Psychosocial Nursing

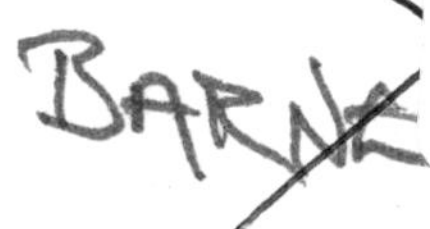

This volume is sponsored by
the Cassel Bursary Trust

Psychosocial Nursing

edited by

ELIZABETH BARNES

TAVISTOCK PUBLICATIONS
London · New York · Sydney · Toronto · Wellington

First published in 1968
by Tavistock Publications Limited
11 New Fetter Lane, London EC4
First published as a Social Science Paperback in 1968
Printed in Great Britain
in 11 pt Imprint
by Cox and Wyman Limited
Fakenham, Norfolk

S.B.N. *422 73010 6*

Distributed in the USA by Barnes and Noble Inc.

This volume, comprising papers written over the period 1946 to 1967, has been compiled as a tribute to
T. F. MAIN, M.D., D.P.M.,
medical director of the Cassel Hospital

Contents

PART III · FAMILY-CENTRED NURSING (1956–1966)

PART IV · APPLICATION OF PSYCHOSOCIAL NURSING

PART V · SUMMING UP

Foreword

This collection of papers is a very good way of paying a compliment to Dr T. F. Main on the completion of twenty-one years as medical director of the Cassel Hospital. It has given me great pleasure to be asked to write a brief foreword.

In fact, there is little need for any such to be written, for the papers explain themselves very well. They give insight into Dr Main's work and demonstrate some of the reasons for the considerable effectiveness of the pioneer effort that the Cassel Hospital still continues.

I was one of the small original staff of the Tavistock Clinic in London when it started in 1920. It was, and still is, primarily concerned with outpatients, though it had a residential centre for some time. Earlier, I had some experience of the work of Bowden House, a residential home for psychoneurotic patients. When the Cassel Hospital was inaugurated in 1919, therefore, I was naturally interested, and happy when I was asked at a later stage to serve on the medical advisory committee. Under its early directors the Cassel did good steady work, providing the kind of psychotherapy now considered conventional. Its story over the past twenty-one years is one of innovation, dominated by psycho-analysis and imaginative organizational thinking.

In 1946, I was one of the small selection group that offered the directorship to Dr Main. I knew him well. For some years he had been a colleague in the Royal Army Medical Corps during the Second World War. After various jobs in Home Command and in the Middle East, he was given full responsibility and charge of advising on all psychiatric activities for the British 2nd and Canadian 3rd Armies in Europe. For a relatively short time after, he went to Northfield Military Hospital, near Birmingham, the Army's largest and somewhat experimental mental hospital. Here he began to show his capacity for new conceptions in psychiatry and of the doctor–patient relationship, opening up the road for all such work in civil hospitals. It is not only that group therapy began to come into its own at Northfield; the concept of the therapeutic community developed, and has now spread to hospitals in the United Kingdom, North America, and many other areas of the world.

This process of creating and working on new ideas has been carried through at the Cassel Hospital, an example to mental health workers all over the world. Running through the whole of Dr Main's work has been the idea of the psychiatric team, and this is well illustrated by the publication of this book of papers written by medical and nursing members of the hospital staff.

Naturally, the process necessitated much changing of outlook, by both medical and nursing personnel, but it has paid handsomely, as it does whenever it is properly applied. At the Cassel, no doors are closed to exploration. Work with mothers and babies, and with families generally, is described in some of these papers. It is important to note the wise use of psycho-analytic principles in all these developments, though relatively few inpatients have been able to have more than the beginnings of a personal analysis.

My congratulations and gratitude to the authors will be shared by all who read this fascinating collection of their experiences. Above all, I congratulate Tom Main himself for the friendly leadership and the courageous use of the team and of his very intelligent imagination.

J. R. Rees
London, 1968

Introduction

The papers that follow, many by nurses who have benefited from the Cassel Bursary Trust, deserve some account of the history that led up to them, especially since the Trust has sponsored this publication.

As one of the original Trustees, and at present chairman, I am privileged to be able to record sincere thanks to various organizations and individuals who have made this experience possible to selected nurses.

The Trust was founded in 1942 by Sir Felix Cassel, Bt., with the object of interesting nurses in the neuroses (the term generally used at the time) and in the work of the Cassel Hospital, founded by his uncle, Sir Ernest Cassel, Bt., in 1919. Sir Felix would, I believe, have been gratified to know the outcome of his generosity and keen interest in nursing. He always insisted that the Trust should be independent of the hospital, though the scholars were to study subjects allied to its work and part of the first courses included practical work in the hospital.

The scholarships that the Trust provided for senior nurses, though most valuable, could affect only a very limited number and, as the years went by and with the advent of Dr T. F. Main as medical director of the hospital and adviser to the Trust, a much wider picture of the mental health field came into view. The Trust sponsored summer schools, conferences, seminars, and teaching groups, which enabled more nurses to become aware of current problems and ways of thinking about them.

The pioneer nature of the hospital was reflected in the outlook of the members of the Trust. With the introduction of the national health service in 1948 the needs of the community were brought to light more forcibly, as also was the reaction of the staff to change. Carefully thought-out changes in the organization of the hospital to meet the needs of patients demonstrated the possibility not only of reducing the number of staff required for various grades but of marked financial savings. The continuing study of the doctor–nurse–patient relationship, of who is doing what to whom and why, makes it possible to clarify changing roles and relationships as they are affected by changes among staff and patients. Each new member, patient or staff, has something valuable to teach and to learn in the hospital community.

The thinking of the World Health Organization and the British Ministry of Health influenced the Trust. From suggestions made by WHO, the Ministry encouraged the summer schools and courses for ward sisters, public health nurses, nurse tutors, matrons, and midwives as desirable experiments worthy of support.

Throughout these years, the chairman and members of the Cassel Hospital Management Committee recognized the potential of individual members of the nursing staff and made it possible for them to undertake work of an unusual nature. To mention a few of the beneficiaries of this far-sighted policy: Elizabeth Barnes, who edits this book, was enabled to use the opportunity provided by the *Nursing Times* to study journalism, and subsequently became co-ordinator of an international study of psychological problems in general hospitals (Barnes, 1961). Eileen Skellern was seconded to the Royal College of Nursing to undertake research into the role of the ward sister; her report is reprinted in Part IV of this book. Gillian Elles worked as tutor at the Cassel while also being sister-in-charge of the psychiatric outpatient department at St Bartholomew's Hospital, London; she was seconded to undertake an investigation into the costs of neurotic illness, reported in Chapter 12.

The unusual situation of having a part-time matron for a period (1958–63) enabled Doreen Weddell to train as a child psycho-analyst after she qualified as an associate member of the British Psycho-Analytical Society. This venture was supported by the South West Metropolitan Regional Hospital Board and by the Ministry of Health. At the time, it was felt that this experiment in the particular circumstances would have possible rewards for the national health service as a whole. This book is some justification of that idea. Miss Weddell, as matron, was formally responsible for teaching. Her papers, therefore, show the importance of educational principles in theory and practice as applied to psychiatric nursing.

Throughout these experiments, the late Hon. Dr Walter

Maclay, psychiatric adviser to the Ministry of Health, gave sympathetic understanding and valuable advice which we greatly appreciated.

Personal thanks are due to the Ministry of Health for allowing me to remain a member of the Trust while Chief Nursing Officer, MOH, and for the experience I had as a member of the Government Working Party on the Recruitment and Training of Nurses (1946) and of two WHO conferences on nursing (1953–6), all of which contributed to my understanding of the importance of what the Cassel Hospital was trying to do. These experiences also served to make me an ardent advocate of experimental schemes that might affect nursing and individual nurses. The value of statutory and voluntary bodies co-ordinating their efforts is demonstrated in these papers.

It was the Cassel nurses who first proposed to mark Dr Main's twenty-one years as medical director with this collection of papers, an idea that the Trust gladly agreed to sponsor. It is proof, I think, of how much the nurses value Dr Main's teaching and his interest and help in their understanding and care of patients with psychiatric disturbances. I hope these papers will help other nurses to share something of the pleasure, pain, and excitement of these twenty-one years and of the continuing endeavour to increase knowledge and skill during the next twenty years or so.

The purpose of this introduction is to try to show how a small voluntary Trust can have far-reaching effects on nursing education in group dynamics, teamwork, and the study of changing attitudes, all of which bring direct benefit to patients. So often we think of new studies being filed away without action. These papers show that there are exceptions.

Elizabeth Cockayne
London, 1968

List of Contributors

BERTA ANDRATSCHKE, M.D., assistant medical director (1960–5) and former acting deputy, the Cassel Hospital.

ELIZABETH BARNES, S.R.N., former ward sister, the Cassel Hospital; matron, the Henderson Hospital (1961–5); tutor, King's Fund College of Hospital Management.

ELIZABETH COCKAYNE, D.B.E., S.R.N., S.C.M., former chief nursing officer, Ministry of Health; chairman, the Cassel Bursary Trust.

HAZEL EDWARDS, S.R.N., former ward sister, superintendent of nursing (1963–6), the Cassel Hospital; tutor, King's Fund College of Hospital Management.

GILLIAN W. ELLES, S.R.N., S.C.M., former ward sister and tutor, the Cassel Hospital; tutor, King's Fund College of Hospital Management; associate member, British Psycho-Analytical Society.

E. JEANETTE GAZDAR, S.R.N., S.C.M., former ward sister, present catering officer, the Cassel Hospital.

IRENE GLEESON, S.R.N., former ward sister, the Cassel Hospital.

THOMAS FORREST MAIN, M.D., D.P.M., medical director, the Cassel Hospital; associate member, British Psycho-Analytical Society.

DOREEN MARTIN, S.R.N., S.C.M., M.T.D., former ward sister, present matron, the Cassel Hospital.

JOHN R. REES, C.B.E., M.D., F.R.C.P., D.P.H., former director, World Federation for Mental Health; member, the Cassel Hospital Management Committee.

JOAN RUSH, S.R.N., S.C.M., former ward sister, the Cassel Hospital; tutor, King's Fund College of Hospital Management.

C. G. M. SCHODT, S.R.N., former ward sister, the Cassel Hospital.

EILEEN SKELLERN, S.R.N., R.M.N., S.T.D., former ward sister, the Cassel Hospital; former sister-in-charge, Social Rehabilitation Unit, Belmont Hospital (renamed Henderson Hospital); present superintendent of nursing, the Bethlem Royal and Maudsley Hospitals.

JANICE WEBSTER, S.R.N., R.M.N., former ward sister, the Cassel Hospital; present matron, Henderson Hospital.

DOREEN WEDDELL, S.R.N., S.C.M., former matron, the Cassel Hospital (1946–63); associate member, British Psycho-Analytical Society.

BLODWEN WIGLEY, S.R.N., R.F.N., former ward sister and deputy matron, the Cassel Hospital.

Editorial Note

The five parts of this book present the lines of thought and study pursued at the Cassel Hospital, and subsequent changes in its therapeutic organization and in the training of its nurses.

Part I begins with the paper written in 1946 in which T. F. Main first introduced the term 'therapeutic community', the concept from which subsequent developments sprang. There follow a concise historical account of the hospital itself and an outline of the training course for nurses.

The many opportunities for learning provided for nurses by patients is the dominant theme of the next two parts. Part II shows how the theory and practice of psychosocial nursing evolved through painstaking study of the patient–doctor–nurse relationship. It includes an account of the first steps to involve families in the treatment of their sick members and in the life of the hospital community, a practice bringing further changes in the nurses' work, as described more fully in Part III.

Big changes in the nursing profession and in the organization of hospitals followed the introduction of the national health service during the years covered by this book. Part IV demonstrates the application of psychosocial nursing techniques in these wider fields.

The final part is short. Doreen Weddell's paper, 'Change as a Learning Situation', well serves as a summary to all that has gone before.

The contributors and the editorial committee join the editor in recording their thanks to all those who, each in his special way and at different times, made this publication possible. The debt to patients can be but inadequately acknowledged, and behind each paper is the work of many colleagues – medical, nursing, administrative, and domestic – who have been remembered as the papers have been compiled. To them, to the Cassel Hospital Management Committee, and the Cassel Bursary Trust, gratitude is now expressed.

A special acknowledgement is due to the secretaries who, over the years, have grappled uncomplainingly with illegible handwriting, incoherent tape-recordings, and elusive references, during the drafting and redrafting of these papers.

Bringing together twenty-eight papers written by fourteen authors during a time-span of twenty-one years presents no small editorial problem. The editor wishes personally to thank the authors and all the above people who helped to make the task easier. One thing only made it possible: the editor has shared with the authors, and many other colleagues whose names do not appear in these pages, the fun, heartache, and pride of learning and working at the Cassel Hospital.

Elizabeth Barnes
London, 1968

Acknowledgements

Permission given by the following publishers, journals, and organizations to reproduce published material is gratefully acknowledged:

The Association of Hospital Matrons, for 'Some Aspects of Personality Development' by Doreen Weddell, a paper read at the Association's annual general meeting, 1955.

The *British Journal of Medical Psychology*, London, for 'The Ailment' by T. F. Main, an address from the chair to the Medical Section, British Psychological Society, 1957, published in Vol. 30, Part 3, pp. 129–145 (1957).

The *Bulletin of the Menninger Clinic*, Topeka, Kansas, for 'The Hospital as a Therapeutic Institution' by T. F. Main, published in Vol. 10, pp. 66–70 (1946).

The Cassel Hospital Management Committee, for the Medical Director's Report on 'Selection of Nurses', from the Cassel Hospital *Medical and General Reports* for the year ending 31 December 1946; and for the Minutes of a Patients' Meeting, from the Cassel Hospital *Reports* for the five years 1 April 1953 to 31 March 1958.

The *Davidson Clinic Bulletin*, Edinburgh, for 'A Fragment on Mothering' by T. F. Main (1958).

The *International Journal of Nursing Studies*, Oxford, for 'Changing Hospital Attitudes' by Elizabeth Barnes, published in Vol. 1, pp. 11–16 (1963); and for extracts from 'Nursing Families in a Therapeutic Community' by Janice Webster, published in Vol. 3, pp. 1–7 (1966).

The *International Nursing Review*, London, for extracts from 'Family-centred Nursing' by Doreen Weddell, published in Vol. 8, No. 6, pp. 20–25 (1961); and for 'Change as a Learning Situation' by Doreen Weddell, published in Vol. 12, No. 5 (1965).

International Universities Press, New York, for 'Mothers with Children on a Psychiatric Unit' by T. F. Main, a chapter in *Frontiers in General Hospital Psychiatry* edited by Louis Linn (1961).

The *Nursing Mirror*, London, for extracts from 'Family-centred Nursing' by C. G. M. Schodt, published 25 November 1960.

The *Nursing Times*, London, for extracts from 'The Education of the Nurse' by Doreen Weddell, published 16 September 1955; for 'Human Relations in Nursing Administration' by Doreen Weddell, published 30 December 1955; and for 'Nursing Emotionally Disturbed Patients', a symposium by Doreen Weddell *et al.*, published in May, June, and July 1957, adapted from papers read at the Psychotherapy and Social Psychiatry Section of the Royal Medico-Psychological Association in July 1956.

Psychotherapy and Psychosomatics, Basel, for 'Change as a Learning Situation' by Doreen Weddell, published in Vol. 13, pp. 201–205 (1965).

The Royal College of Nursing, London, for 'The Role of the Ward Sister', a monograph by Eileen Skellern, published in 1953.

PART I

The Hospital as a Therapeutic Institution

Editorial Note

The three papers in Part I present the basic concepts and history of the Cassel Hospital and describe the training of its nurses.

T. F. Main's paper was the first of a symposium written at the special request of Karl Menninger for publication in the *Bulletin of the Menninger Clinic* in 1946. The paper has not dated. Its startling simplicity and sense retain the power to surprise the new reader and set him thinking.

Other contributors to that now famous *Bulletin* were W. R. Bion, Harold Bridger, Susan Davidson, Millicent C. Dewar, and S. H. Foulkes, who, with Dr Main and others, were working at the Northfield Military Hospital. Their combined imagination and experimentation in the treatment of mental breakdown in soldiers during the Second World War were radically to change treatment methods and the internal organization of mental hospitals in the coming years.

The Cassel Hospital itself, however, sprang from the terrible stress and waste of the First World War, as Berta Andratschke recounts in the second paper. A valued member of the staff for many years, she helped to initiate many of the changes she describes.

The new concept of the purpose of a hospital demanded nursing of a different order. Doreen Weddell gives the conceptual framework, planning, and practice of a training which she has guided since it began and which changed with the changing needs of the hospital and the community it serves. Prepared and given at the request of the medical staff in 1961, her paper needed little editing to bring the description up to date.

1 · *The Hospital as a Therapeutic Institution*

BY T. F. MAIN[1]

By tradition a hospital is a place wherein sick people may receive shelter from the stormy blasts of life, the care and attention of nursing and medical auxiliaries, and the individual attention of a skilled doctor. The concept of a hospital as a refuge too often means, however, that patients are robbed of their status as responsible human beings. Too often they are called 'good' or 'bad' only according to the degree of their passivity in the face of the hospital's demand for their obedience, dependency, and gratitude. The fine traditional mixture of charity and discipline they receive is a practised technique for removing their initiative as adult beings, and making them 'patients'. They are less trouble, thus, to the staff. Hospitals that follow this orthodoxy are usually designed for the individual treatment of the individual patient by an individual doctor, not in a real social setting, but in a state of retirement from society. So, isolated and dominated, the patient tends to remain gripped by the hospital machine even in the games or prescribed occupations which occupy his time between treatments.

Within such a setting, health and stability are too often bought at the excessive price of desocialization. Sooner or later the patient, alone and unsupported, must face the difficult task of returning to the society in which he became unstable, there to regain social integration and a daily sense of values and purpose. This task is no light one for a desocialized man, however healthy he may have become.

The design of a hospital as a social retreat also ignores positive therapeutic forces – the social support and emotional opportunities that are granted in spontaneously structured communities. It is

[1] Then Lt.-Col., R.A.M.C.

true that radical individual treatment can free the inner drives of the patient and make him capable of full and stable social life, but it fails to give him an assured technique for full social participation – he can learn this only from the impact of society itself. Treatment of the neurotic patient, who suffers from a disturbance of social relationships, cannot therefore be regarded as satisfactory unless it is undertaken within a framework of social reality which can provide him with opportunities for attaining fuller social insight and for expressing and modifying his emotional drives according to the demands of real life. In any case, the fact must be faced that radical individual psychotherapy is not a practicable proposition for the huge numbers of patients confronting the psychiatric world today. It is doubtful whether the hospital can usefully remain a building within which individual treatment is practised. Perhaps it must become a therapeutic institution.

A THERAPEUTIC COMMUNITY

The Northfield Experiment is an attempt to use a hospital not as an organization run by doctors in the interests of their own greater technical efficiency, but as a community with the immediate aim of full participation of all its members in its daily life and the eventual aim of the resocialization of the neurotic individual for life in ordinary society. Ideally, it has been conceived as a therapeutic setting with a spontaneous and emotionally structured (rather than medically dictated) organization in which all staff and patients engage. Any attempt to permit or create such a setting demands tolerance, a willingness to profit by error, and a refusal to jump to conclusions; but certain matters appear to be plain. The daily life of the community must be related to real tasks, truly relevant to the needs and aspirations of the small society of the hospital and the larger society in which it is set; there must be no barriers between the hospital and the rest of society; full opportunity must be available for identifying and analysing the interpersonal barriers that stand in the way of participation in a full community life.

These are not small requirements and they have demanded a review of our attitudes as psychiatrists towards our own status and responsibilities. The anarchical rights of the doctor in the traditional hospital society have to be exchanged for the more sincere role of member in a real community, responsible not only to himself and his superiors, but to the community as a whole, privileged and restricted only in so far as the community allows or demands. He no longer owns 'his' patients. They are given up to the community which is to treat them and which owns them and him. Patients are no longer his captive children, obedient in nursery-like activities, but have sincere adult roles to play, and are free to reach for responsibilities and opinions concerning the community of which they are a part. They, as well as he, must be free to discuss a rationale of daily hospital life, to identify and analyse the problems, formulate the conditions and forge the enthusiasms of group life. The patients must be free to plan and organize activities of actual hospital procedure and thus face together problems of immediate social reality. Failures of organization, internal problems of apathy, insecurity, and hostility, as well as ordinary practical difficulties, are matters for solution by the patients who own the community and create the problems.

THE PSYCHIATRIST'S ROLE

Sometimes because he is an ordinary community member, often because of his special knowledge, the psychiatrist's opinion is sought when difficulties arise. He may attempt resolution of the interpersonal tensions creating the difficulty, by group therapy within a functional or a reflective group, or may only identify the emotional difficulties involved and leave the solution to the patients. But he does not seek *ex cathedra* status. Indeed, he must refuse any platform offered to him and abrogate his usual right to pass judgement on intergroup claims or problems. The psychiatrist has to tolerate disorder and tension up to the point when it is plain that the community itself must tackle these as problems of group life. In the case of individual behaviour (for example, in men with depression) he may have to wait for a social regression to be worked through and for spontaneous reparative drives to make their appearance, or for the patient to ask for insight into his disturbance or behaviour.

The psychiatrist is ready to redefine a practical problem in terms of attitudes or relationships, to reorientate another, to illumine a third, and in a fourth to act as a catalyst for social response and awareness. His role as a technician among, rather than a superintendent of, his patients certainly does not mean that he can remain inactive. He should be a sincere commentator and participant in many of the social fields that wax and wane with the varying needs of the fluid population of the hospital, and be prepared to create conditions for the exercise of growing drives and interests or to open channels of communication between certain social groupings. He should be active in providing opportunities for therapeutic intercourse between patients and in modifying the practical barriers of time and geography standing in the way of this. His daily work is to study and facilitate the growth of the social pull and push which allows the isolate to expand in social integration to the therapeutic end of rich social and industrial life relating to the real community in which the hospital is set.

It must be pointed out that the medical man, educated to play a grandiose role among the sick, finds it difficult to renounce his power, to shoulder social responsibilities in a hospital, and to grant sincerely to his patients independence and adulthood. But it is no easier for the rest of the staff. It is difficult to live in a field undergoing internal stress without wanting to trade upon authority and crush the spontaneity that gives rise to the stress, to demand dependence and to impose law and order from above. Such measures, however, do not solve the problem of neurosis in social life, but are a means of evading the issue.

RELATIONS OF THE STAFF

The members of the staff, too, have their problems, their fear, so to say, of the social id, and they have their own emotional needs. Group discussions held about specific problems, among those who are involved by them, the exposure of the individual to social sanction and pressure in group meetings of patients and staff discussing matters relating to their daily work, are necessary to prevent the growth of the barriers that exist between patients and staff in most hospitals. The nursing staff, the kitchen and administrative staffs, the social therapy staff, the psychiatrists, the patients, all have sectional and interrelated problems in immediate practical fields and involving interpersonal and intergroup tensions. The granting of social significance and effect to the daily lives of the staff and their integration with the whole hospital community and its purpose, in general and in detail, are helped by routine meetings and social occasions, and by participation in group therapeutic sessions. Apart from the resultant increase in sincerity and social health gained by the extension of the social boundaries of the staffs within the hospital, the effect on 'atmosphere' is very important. And only thus can the whole community engage continuously upon its aim of adapting to the needs and problems of its participants.

INDIVIDUAL NEEDS

Attention to the hospital as a therapeutic community does not, of course, preclude attention to the individual problems of its members. Rather, with the recognition of the legitimate aspirations of others, an increasing provision is freely made by the community for individual limitations and needs. One group of patients, who called themselves 'The Co-ordination Group', set up office and prepared to cater on demand to needs in real life which were not provided otherwise by the hospital; they specialized in unusual requests, and in seeking out jobs to suit a patient or in seeking patients to do certain jobs.

Again, the psychiatrist will give individual attention to those whose problems are not being satisfactorily solved within the various therapeutic social fields created in the hospital. The man whose social capacity is too low to allow him participation in a group activity even of 'low tension' is free to choose solitary activities; and where his desire is to avoid society and activity, he will be given a single room and permitted to do nothing. For despite the basic conviction that it is no part of the function of a hospital to compel a compulsory retreat from society in exchange for treatment for all those who enter its doors, there are many patients whose best immediate relationship with society is isolation, dependency, or personal regression.

Northfield provides facilities to meet these occasions: men mourning the loss of their comrades in battle are given full facilities to carry out this social task; a darkened ward and continuous narcosis are available for those who express themselves by symbolic illness as being in need of a period of infantile behaviour; the man with problems of aggression may be granted a job involving satisfactions for his aggression; and the cynical may receive the support of the personal transference situation until he is able to accept life in a small group of chosen friends. When acute needs have been satisfied, however, these patients are faced with a wide range of social and industrial opportunities, and are free to move at their own choice and at their own speed within the social fields that best suit them. As every social field is connected by emotional channels with others, the patient thus embarks upon life in a real society which can continue, up to a limit, to allow him an expansion of his social relationships. This limit is not set by hospital boundaries, for he may work and form relationships within the wider geographic boundaries set by modern forms of travel.

THE AIM

The socialization of neurotic drives, their modification by social demands within a real setting, the ego-strengthening, the increased capacity for sincere and easy social relationships, the socialization of superego demands, provide the individual with a capacity and a technique for stable life in a real role in the real world. The common remark made when a patient is asked on leaving why he is better, is a vague, 'I don't know why. I found something that suited me. Then I met some nice people. I think that helped.' The psychiatrist is rarely mentioned as a therapeutic agent. When he is highly praised, it is regarded as a failure of therapy. For, with increasing social and industrial vectors from the larger society outside the hospital there should be no regrets on leaving; rather an increased zest for life and confidence that the problems it presents can be met and faced without inefficiency or unhappiness.

2 · *The Changing Face of a Hospital*[1]

BY BERTA ANDRATSCHKE

The Cassel Hospital, founded in 1919, was one of several pioneer adventures in medicine promoted by Sir Ernest Cassel, Bt. Having been greatly impressed with the treatment of so-called 'shell-shock' at Seale Hayne Military Hospital, Devon, Sir Ernest decided to endow and equip a hospital for civilian patients suffering from functional nervous disorders similar to those he had seen in soldiers returning from the trenches in the First World War. Patients treated in the new hospital were to be drawn from the educated population and would be expected to pay towards their treatment according to their means.

The first medical director, Dr T. A. Ross, was originally a general practitioner with a natural 'feel' for nervous ailments (Ross, 1923), who had already made a name as a successful therapist of shell-shock. The hospital, the first of its kind in the United Kingdom, quickly became known throughout the country and abroad. The changes in its organization reflect changes in concepts of the neuroses and in the social and economic conditions of the country.

Originally situated in a large country house, Swaylands, near Penshurst, Kent, with eighty acres of garden and parkland, the hospital now faces a village common, but backs on to an aircraft factory. At first the patients' day was planned by the staff and their material needs were catered for by thirty housemaids. The patients went to bed on admission and the traditional bedside doctor–patient relationship was at once established. Meals were a social event and everyone dressed for dinner. Now the housemaids have

[1] Adapted from a paper read at the Third World Congress of Psychiatry, Montreal, 1961.

gone and the patients clean up and cook their own meals as they do at home. Social events were arranged by occupational therapists. The last left nearly twenty years ago and patients now find their own amusements and occupations outside and use their initiative in helping to run the hospital.

Neuroses in the early years were attributed by many to biochemical changes, nose and sinus infections, intestinal poison, and other such conditions. The most popular diagnosis was neurasthenia, followed by depression and anxiety neurosis. Empirical procedures, suggestion, persuasion, and hypnosis were used.

Many patients improved and remained well, as the early medical reports show. Some patients who failed to improve in hospital reported great improvement soon after discharge when treated by other doctors. This led Dr Ross to the study of transference and to a more dynamic approach to therapy (Ross, 1932, 1936). By 1935 the first psycho-analyst had been appointed.

Dr Ross retired and was followed by Dr E. W. Anderson, who resigned a year later. Dr C. H. Rogerson was appointed medical director in 1937 at the age of twenty-seven, just over a year after he had first drawn attention to the link between hay fever, anxiety, and high intelligence in children (Rogerson, Hardcastle & Duguid, 1935). He guided the hospital through the Second World War, resigning in 1946 to work at the Seton Institute, Baltimore, where he died two years later.

The hospital was evacuated when the air raids increased to a quiet country hotel in the Midlands, with room for thirty civilian patients. Swaylands was taken over by the War Office. Both staff and patients caught the wartime urgency. There was work to be done, firewood to be cut, grassland to plough, vegetables to grow; help was needed on nearby farms, in canteens, and in nurseries. The medical staff was reduced to two. Pressure on beds and a growing waiting-list made it essential to seek time-saving methods. Although dynamic psychotherapy remained the important treatment, the new physical methods were introduced and used for a short period and it was at this time that group therapy was first employed.

Dr T. F. Main became medical director in October 1946. Treatment continued on the same lines at first. Psychodrama enjoyed a short vogue. More requests for admission came and the search for a new home became urgent. Swaylands was still being used by the military.

An eighteenth-century house overlooking Ham Common, Richmond, Surrey, was bought towards the end of 1947, and is the hospital's present site. Many difficulties were faced, the noise of a host of workmen, the recruiting of new staff of all grades. The resulting confusion and tension were dealt with then, as they still are, by group discussion of staff and patients and joint consultation among the various staff groups.

Six months later saw the advent of the national health service, which guaranteed medical care, including hospital treatment, to every citizen. Increased cost of living made private treatment prohibitive to all but the rich, and long-term stay in a private hospital became too expensive for the kinds of patients for whom the hospital was originally meant. The decision to join the new service was taken by the management committee after the chairman, Sir Felix Cassel, had received assurance from the Ministry of Health that the hospital's psychotherapeutic service, unique in the United Kingdom, would be continued and that the hospital would remain a national one, drawing its patients from the whole country.

By 1948 the orientation of the hospital, with the new medical appointments, was entirely psycho-analytic. Difficulties of inpatient analysis were now brought to light. The analyst could not easily remain a detached figure seen only in the consulting room; he was a member of a hospital staff involved in the management of patients. Our early struggles with this problem show three distinct phases.

At first, the analysts took over the management of each other's patients, an arrangement that created complicated medical relationships to the detriment of treatment. The second phase was the development in 1952 of a social therapy unit, STU, with a staff of psychiatrist, nurses, and social worker, who took full charge of the general management of patients, their daily life, drugs, occupations, rehabilitation. The analyst no longer saw his patients outside the consulting room. The STU staff and the analysts stayed in their own roles and had no consultation. At first this arrangement worked well, but dissatisfaction spread as the analysts began to disagree with STU decisions and the STU staff criticized the analysts' handling of their patients. Both sides were poorly informed because they did not communicate and relied on the patients for information. Things were further complicated in that a few patients had private analysts outside the hospital, a practice later prohibited by the national health service regulations. This second phase was abandoned in 1954.

In the third phase, the STU remained but the analysts and STU doctor had regular communication. Information on the patient's performance in hospital was given to the analyst concerned, and he in turn could advise on, but not order, management. This was a deviation from the usual analytic requirement but it highlighted many hitherto unrecognized problems of the long-stay patients, the dependency created, the secondary gains, and the increased problem of rehabilitation. This third phase lasted only one year.

We then decided not to admit patients for psycho-analysis unless they could become outpatients in a short time. Most patients now had psycho-analytically oriented psychotherapy, individually or in groups; physical methods of treatment had long been abandoned. During this time a few patients were treated by a colleague, the late Dr S. S. Davidson, by the Rosen technique of direct analysis.

The medical organization was divided into semi-autonomous units, each with its own group of patients, doctors, and nurses. Each medical unit became responsible for its own area of the building, including cleaning and decorating, for decisions on the treatment and general management of its own group, and for providing some community service for the hospital. One unit, for example, took over the dining-room service. In the course of time, as domestic and maintenance staff left, they were not replaced – a deliberate policy to provide patients with real opportunities for work and housekeeping responsibilities. Basically a therapeutic measure, this policy also happened to result in financial savings.

The practice of admitting mothers and children began in 1948 when a mother asked if she could bring in her small son because there was no one at home to look after him. Our attitude changed over the years from allowing the admission of children to recommending it, and eventually almost to insisting on it. Husbands were encouraged to spend weekends with their wives and children if the latter could not go home.

In 1958 we halved the bed numbers and freed the medical staff to undertake more outpatient service, the treatment of choice for many patients. The outpatients, drawn mainly from the neighbourhood, helped us to set down roots in the local community. At the same time, we were beginning to develop closer contact with the professional community, particularly those groups with wide contacts, such as public health nurses, probation officers, general practitioners, and medical officers of health, for whom seminars were arranged.

Changes in treatment and management through these years – from regression to self-reliance, from rest and refuge to activity, from struggling with the conscious mind to studying the unconscious, from isolation to family and community contact – have demanded new ways of thinking for staff and patients. The constant search goes on to develop and improve our methods of helping patients to regain and maintain their responsible adult status. The basic medical policy, laid down by the hospital's founder and followed by each medical director, remains unchanged, however: intensive study, staff training, research, and the treatment of patients who can benefit from psychotherapy.

3 · *Outline of Nurse Training*

BY DOREEN WEDDELL

Originally, the nursing staff of the Cassel Hospital consisted of assistant nurses, with one or two trained nurses and a matron; but no mention is made of them in the early hospital brochures.

The first formal training, started in 1941, was an eighteen months' course for ward sisters interested in nursing patients with neurotic disturbances. The interest shown in this course by general hospital nurses led the late Sir Felix Cassel to institute the Cassel Bursary Trust,[1] which provided a shorter course of four months for senior nurses who, it was hoped, would then be able to bring a psychological approach to the nursing of patients in general hospitals. Most of these early students were to become well known in the nursing world.

Since 1948, when the last of these courses were held, the hospital has offered two kinds of training: short intensive courses for nurses of various grades and fields, and a longer course for nurses of ward-sister status. The intention of both types of course was to feed back into the nursing profession experiences gained while working in the Cassel Hospital, particularly the understanding of patients as individuals and of their interaction in a family and as groups in the hospital community.

The courses have always been based on the work of Freud. The first book the Bursary students read was *The Interpretation of Dreams* (Freud, 1900). In 1946 *The Psychopathology of Everyday Life* (Freud, 1914) became the nurses' textbook, joined two years later by Klein and Riviere's *Love, Hate and Reparation* (1936). At that time one of the main training tasks was to convince the nurses of the reality of the unconscious. In the present day we can

[1] See Introduction, p. xii – Ed.

assume that the nurses recognize this or they would not apply for training.

SHORT COURSES

The first summer school was held in 1949, financed by the Trust, and was attended by thirty ward sisters from general and children's hospitals and by a few nurse tutors. The broad theme of the school was 'The Development of Human Behaviour in the Family and Society', and a number of experts spoke on their specialties: Miss Anna Freud on the meaning of illness to children; Dr John Bowlby on the child's capacity to form relationships; Dr A. T. M. Wilson on the hospital and the community; and Dr Main on hospitalization and reactions to illness. All these lectures were followed by group discussion, a practice still continued although the design of the schools has changed as our experience has grown.

By the next year the General Nursing Council had introduced psychology into its syllabus. We adopted this new syllabus as the basis of teaching for subsequent summer schools and an amplified version of it has been used for the longer training course since that time.

In the summer schools of 1955, 1956, and 1966, more intensive use was made of senior nurses in the Cassel Hospital, who were now trained to take the group discussions and had learned to understand current group anxieties. The groups' anxieties were reported back to the speaker concerned, who would then try to deal with them in such a way as to reduce the anxiety and produce a useful learning situation. For example, in the group discussions following one lecture we found that the students were so curious about the speaker and his interests and background that this aspect had to be dealt with before further learning could occur. Similarly, when towards the end of the first week there was to be a change of speaker, the students' concern about the loss of someone they knew and the prospect of adjusting to a stranger was shown in their preoccupation with topics such as promiscuity, adoption, and death. In dealing with these topics it was possible to relate the students' current feelings to the way in which children feel and, through children, to their own nursing of patients in the wards. In these later schools, only speakers who could work in this particular way with the Cassel nurses were chosen.

Experiences gained in the summer schools have been fed back both into teaching methods used in the longer courses and into practical nursing techniques in the hospital.

WARD SISTERS' COURSE IN PSYCHOLOGICAL NURSING

When the hospital had settled in its new home after the Second World War,[1] the longer course of one year was redesigned and a more careful selection procedure instituted.[2] Lectures and seminars, given mainly by medical staff, covered all aspects of emotional development and psychopathology, and the matron held discussions on nursing problems, general administration, and the organizational design of the hospital.

Nurses were given a great deal of psychopathological information, of little practical use, some personally disturbing. While both the doctors and the nurses were pleased with their academic achievements, considerable confusion of roles between doctors and nurses became a dominant feature. The nurses' dissatisfaction with their nursing of some patients led to an investigation which altered our whole approach to nursing. Subsequent teaching and many nursing procedures have been based on the findings.[3]

FAMILY-CENTRED NURSING

Patient assessment has always been an important part of practical training. In 1955 the nurses began to interview prospective patients and their relatives in their own homes. The training course was again redesigned and given a new name, family-centred nursing, the intention being that the nurses would now spend a considerable amount of their time with patients and relatives at home. The hospital chauffeur taught the nurses to drive, and there were seminars on family interviewing. The new skills developed alongside the increasing tendency to admit husbands, wives, and children to the hospital as complete families.[4]

TRAINING FRAMEWORK

What can be taught and how it should be taught have always been adjusted to the needs of the training group at the time. Sometimes

[1] See Chapter 2 – Ed. [2] See Chapter 23 – Ed.
[3] See Chapters 4, 5, and 6 – Ed. [4] See Part III – Ed.

the greater part of the year will be spent talking about aspects of child development; sometimes this subject will be covered in three or four months. With other groups more time may be needed on the physical manifestations of emotional disturbance. Always the nurses are expected to read around the topic and to answer questions and raise difficulties in discussion. They must, therefore, be moderately intelligent as well as moderately stable.

The basic nursing assumption is the concept that the patient is primarily responsible to himself for himself; the hospital offers certain facilities – living accommodation, medical services, nursing care of a special kind – but how the patient uses these is his own affair. The nurse can help him only in so far as he seeks or can accept help. She will comment on and discuss with him how he makes use of the hospital but, by and large, decisions on such matters will come from him rather than from the nurse. She will work with him on ordinary domestic chores. She will try to verbalize for the patient, if he is unable to, what he is doing in his relationships, and perhaps point out what may be the consequences of his actions, in social and not psychological terms.

A hospital is a peculiar place, quite unlike a normal living arrangement. It is useful to the staff as a means of livelihood, but, for patients, the need for hospital admission may be thought of as an illness in itself which requires treatment. The patient is a member of his family, with a place there and in society of far greater importance to him than anything the hospital can provide. The nurse, therefore, has to learn how to ensure that the hospital's administrative procedures and her own relationship with the patient interfere as little as possible with his relationships at home, with friends, and in society. In general, the patient will spend more time with his family and less in the hospital.

The nurse is expected to understand something of the patient's feelings and phantasies which make him behave as he does, to be aware of her own response to him in varying situations, and to describe this, sometimes to the patient, usually to the doctors and other nurses. She must be able to distinguish between the patient's social anxieties expressed in working relationships, medical unit meetings, and other social situations, and his personal emotional response to certain situations.

She is expected to learn how to be a group member and how to lead a group, seeking to understand the tensions and anxieties the group may be expressing. The nurse's understanding of what is happening in a small group or in the larger hospital community has varied over the years, depending to some extent on the medical staff's interest in such skills.

The nurse must be able to examine and criticize her own and other nurses' techniques freely with her colleagues, without blame or scapegoating, and to adapt and change her techniques as occasion demands. She has to learn to tolerate what at first seems to be chaos, in a situation with little routine work. She will often feel unneeded by patients. She has to accept that what a patient feels and says about her will be coloured by his particular emotional needs and background and may not necessarily have to do with her as a person.

She is responsible to the doctor with whom she works and will carry out his instructions, keeping him informed of all her work with patients when he requests this. As a member of the nursing team she will make observations on and help to develop procedures for nursing and management in conjunction with medical techniques, though such procedures may not necessarily be initiated by the doctors. She is expected to write reports on patients individually and in group situations and such other reports as the medical staff may require.

If the patient is to be regarded as a reasonably responsible person, not unlike the nurse, so the nurse must have opportunity to express herself and to develop her own personality. Her hospital work is only one part of her life.

FORMAL EDUCATION

The new nurse's introduction to the hospital is considered to be very important. What she is expected to do when she first comes is designed with care. She will be introduced personally to all the heads of departments and their staff. She will discuss with the matron the organizational structure of the hospital and its administration, not as a thing in itself but as a setting for nursing patients and for such nursing procedures as may be necessary.

No lectures are given. Emotional development, the foundation of theoretical training, is taught by discussion of the nurse's current experiences with the children in the hospital. Thus the children are helped as the nurse's understanding of their emotional upsets is increased.

There are weekly discussions on interview techniques, and on methods of assessment and evaluation (including report-writing) of work groups, the children's play group, and other social situations in the hospital. There is also daily discussion on the problems of individual patients and children, on group situations and community problems, and on nursing procedures and more general matters. Much of this discussion can be shared with patients.[1] Discussion is dovetailed with experiences in current practical work and may occur at nursing report-time or in nursing meetings or unit meetings.

PRACTICAL WORK

Each nurse is attached to a medical unit for practical training, the senior nurse being responsible for seeing that she gets relevant experience. She carries a case-load of about twelve patients, according to her experience and capability. She has opportunity to nurse patients for individual doctors, for several doctors, individually or as a group. She works with patients in groups, participates in admission procedures, interviews relatives, and does home visits. She observes children in various situations and is expected to understand something of what they express in play. She works with mothers who have their children in hospital and helps husbands to maintain their place in the family. She seeks the co-operation of other patients and families in looking after particularly ill patients. She will have experience in attending and organizing social functions and will be encouraged to develop her particular skills, on the principle that her interests and those of some, at least, of the patients are likely to be similar.

Initially a new nurse is not left on duty alone. A senior nurse is always on call, if not on duty, for consultation. The new nurse only gives drugs specifically ordered by medical staff. If asked for something unusual by a patient she will seek to understand his real distress and will resort to medical advice and support only when she feels that the patient's anxiety is excessive or that she, the nurse, can stand the anxiety no longer.

[1] See also Chapter 20 – Ed.

EXAMINATIONS

The content of the examination held at the end of the course has varied over the years. Currently, the nurse is expected to produce a report from a patient's assessment period, a report from an interview with relatives, a social report on a unit meeting or activity, and a case-history of a patient she has nursed during the year. There are two, sometimes three, three-hour papers. Questions are asked on emotional development, on social and community relationships in the hospital, and on the nursing role with particular patients and in particular situations. Typical questions are: Think of any patient you have nursed, describe the relationship the patient established with you, how it changed during treatment, how the patient used you and the hospital. What are the patient's relationships with other patients? With his family? What difficulties were foreseen in the assessment period? How did these work out?

The nurse also sees the medical director so that he can assess her capacity to verbalize what she has experienced during the period of training.

SOME OBSERVATIONS

Well-marked mood changes, apparent during the training period, have persisted through the years, in spite of alterations in teaching method and content. The first phase is one of elation and idealization: everything is wonderful, no routine, the chance to be an individual, to kick over the traces. There is, also, anxiety about doing the 'right' thing, matching up to the standard set. A lot of reassurance is required during this time on the line that the nurse can only do what she thinks is best at any given moment. It implies that her ideas of what is best will change during the year and that she will only learn by discussing on every occasion what she did, why she did it, and how others might have dealt with the same situation.

This leads to the next phase, one of increasing depression when it is realized that so many things done in the past could have been done differently. An internal adjustment goes on, with the psychic equivalent of digestion, indigestion, and some vomiting. Then comes a phase of considerable confusion, mingled with depression: 'I shall never learn this. I don't understand anything. Nobody helps, nothing is any good.' Clarification begins to set in as examination time approaches!

Through mourning the loss of old ideals and expectations of herself and others, the nurse develops an increased ability to recognize reality-based needs and the capacities of herself and her patients, and to respond appropriately. A degree of inner freedom is achieved as she becomes less tied to automatic patterns of thought and behaviour. She can begin to move more freely in the role required of her, using what she has learned with intelligence and sensitivity. She can accept people and situations as they are, without abandoning hope of such changes as may be desired. Her inner experience of parting and loss while adjusting to a less dependent relationship with patients, staff, and the hospital, stands her in good stead when she seeks to understand patients' difficulties in similar situations.

Most nurses seem to want to stay a further year before they are assured of their skill and can contribute on an equal footing with their colleagues and the medical staff. In this second year more attention is paid to the development of group techniques, to personnel management, and to administration as a nursing procedure. A broad view of the various medical approaches is gained as the nurse works in different medical units.

It is not always easy to match the needs of the nurse in training, emotionally and practically, with the medical staff's need for nurses to look after patients, but an attempt is made to balance these in order to make the best use of the training opportunities provided in the hospital.

PART II

Development of Nursing Techniques (1946–1956)

Editorial Note

These first ten years saw the fundamental change of concept that was to set the new pattern of training and practice in psychosocial nursing.

Doreen Weddell describes the all-giving mothering role of the nurse, which led the nurses to try, with growing failure, to satisfy insatiable demands from patients and to vie with each other in the attempt to live up to impossible expectations.

T. F. Main shows what happened when a research group of senior nurses met with him to try to discover, through discussion, why some of their most valued and experienced colleagues were breaking under the strain of nursing certain patients who came to be called 'special'. Ernst Freud, attached to the nursing staff at the time, acted as secretary to the group. Their search after the factors causing the distress borne by themselves and their junior colleagues cleared their thinking and led to new principles and procedures. Their work was crucial to the development of all later nursing techniques.

Central to the replanning were painstaking clarification of roles, particularly nursing and medical roles, a reorganization of the training course, and the development of new expectations of the nurse and the patient, which Doreen Weddell outlines. Nurses involved in role changes in other hospitals may find that similar investigations are needed to aid the learning process and subsequent development.

The practical results are described in the succeeding five papers by the nurses who were themselves involved. Hazel Edwards shows how the new patient and the new nurse, sharing a common experience, learn the ways of the hospital. Blodwen Wigley's account of the responsibilities shared by her and the patients in the day-to-day organization of the hospital includes the minutes of a patients' meeting. Jeanette Gazdar takes up the same topic, indicating how the roles of the domestic and catering staff changed as the patients began working with them.

The first home visit undertaken by a nurse, described by Irene Gleeson, was the beginning of what eventually became standard nursing practice in helping patients to remain members of their families. Some problems of leaving hospital, for the patient and for the group he leaves behind, are illustrated by Gillian Elles.

All five papers, together with the two by Doreen Weddell, were read at a meeting of the Psychotherapy and Social Psychiatry Section of the Royal Medico-Psychological Association in July 1956, and subsequently published as a symposium by the *Nursing Times*, May, June, and July 1957. T. F. Main's paper was given as an address from the chair to the Medical Section of the British Psychological Society in March 1957, and published in the *British Journal of Medical Psychology*, Vol. 30, Part 3, 1957, pp. 129–45.

Gillian Elles's second paper, the final chapter in this part, describes her investigation into the costs, in human terms, of neurotic breakdown for the patient, his family, the health service, and the national economy.

The printed word is now the only means of communicating the warmth, pain, and intensity of the learning process shared by the nurses during this significant ten-year period. The nurses' experiences in the second decade, though still as personally painful at times, could grow within a structure giving strength and stability derived from the insights gained in the first.

4 · *Nursing Emotionally Disturbed Patients*

BY DOREEN WEDDELL

ATTEMPTING TO MEET THE PATIENT'S APPARENT NEED

At first the emotionally disturbed patient was thought of as an invalid. It was usual for him to spend part of his time in bed; he was waited on, given hot drinks and sedatives at night, and had his day planned for him. The nursing approach was essentially that of a general hospital. Patients were told when they could get up and when they could go to bed; what drugs, aperients, and food they were to have; and what they were to do during the day. Lights were put out at a certain time at night and the nursing staff always knew where patients were and what they were doing. There were some variations, of course, because patients were encouraged to go out. But the nurse always had to know about it. The patients' beds were in small wards and they could have their own things about. But the nurse's task was essentially active: she helped the patient all the time – supporting, encouraging, setting limited goals, being pleased when the patient achieved them, tolerant and understanding if the patient was unsuccessful.

If (as I thought at the time) emotional difficulties or disturbed personal relationships occurred because of unfortunate experiences in childhood, then the task of the nurse was to be to the patient the kind of parent he had not had. If only the patient could be helped to feel that he was loved, that he meant something to someone, and if his special needs could be understood, the bad experiences need not be repeated – this, I thought, must be the nurse's aim. So the expectation was that the nurse would spend as much time as possible with the patient: where the patient was, there should be the nurse. She would listen to his troubles, give all the care, physical and environmental, that she could. What the patient wanted, that he should have, in so far as the nurse could supply it. If the patient was anxious in the day or could not sleep at night, he should have drugs. If he wanted to go out, the nurse should go with him. An attempt would be made to satisfy every wish, as far as possible.

Up to a point this was a satisfactory situation to the patient and to the nurse. The patient had his dependency needs catered for, there was always someone to whom he could turn, someone he felt to be his own. In effect, however, various regressive phenomena became the order of the day – panic states, temper tantrums, special diets, special drugs. Some patients stayed up half the night and slept half the day, others got up in the middle of the night and had long sessions with the night nurse – but all varieties of behaviour were supposed to be understood and catered for.

For her part, the nurse enjoyed being to the patient this all-understanding, all-giving mother that she herself wished she had had. The patient was her child, for whom she would do everything and mean everything. Special bonds would develop between the nurse and the patient; a particular nurse would feel that she alone really understood a particular patient, that she alone of all the nursing staff could help this patient.

THE DRUG SITUATION

Large quantities of drugs were regularly consumed, both by day and by night. If the patient's doctor was away or if his nurse went on holiday the patient would have sedatives instead.

With certain patients there was always a fight over sedatives. They never felt they had enough and would use all their wiles to get more. One particular patient, a man, was extremely anxious. Great beads of sweat would stand out on his forehead and round his mouth, and he slept very badly. During the day he had barbiturates, four-hourly if necessary. It seemed that he had to have a nurse to sit with him while he went to sleep, and a special nurse had this to do each night. When he seemed asleep and she made a move to go, he would mumble in a drunken, dazed way, 'I'm not asleep'. If the nurse persisted in leaving, there would be a terrible to-do. The patient would fall out of bed, throw things about. He once tore the bookcase off the wall. He would threaten to do something to himself. With cigarettes or sweets, 'just one more, nurse', he would bribe and cajole the nurse either to stay with him or to give him more sedative.

The patient was in great distress and so was the nurse. She would be distracted – on the one hand, feeling that only she could help the patient, and, on the other, that other patients were needing her. If she gave the extra sedative now there would be trouble in the early morning. The duty doctor might have to be called in – sometimes he would feel that *he* must stay with the patient, and in the end even more sedative might be given. All this aroused other patients' envy, with increased disturbance. Why should this patient have all the attention? They too were ill and needed extra sedatives or doctor- or nurse-time. If this was not sufficiently apparent to the staff then it must be demonstrated by similar behaviour.

We had not reckoned, it seemed, with the primitive, all-powerful, greedy wishes that are present in everyone, and can never be satisfied, and that this approach inevitably stimulated particularly strongly in some patients.

FAILURE

Sooner or later a crisis would develop. After the most devoted care the patient would hurt the nurse in some way, or disappoint all her efforts by not getting better. He would make more and more demands that were impossible to meet, and turn against the nurse when she had to refuse something. The patient would inevitably succeed in repeating past difficulties in his relationships. However good the nurse endeavoured to be to the patient, something would eventually happen to make the patient feel her to be as bad as everyone else. Somehow or other the nurse would begin to get fed up with the patient, she would begin to feel she had done her bit and would want to withdraw from the situation. But by this time she was at loggerheads with the other nurses over the patient: she had made them feel useless or irritated with him; only she was competent. This meant that she herself had become isolated and 'special' to the nurses' group. How could she leave the patient to their tender mercies? Or she might vindictively say, 'Well, you just try!' The nurse would feel guilty about failing in her task, angry with herself and the patient, in despair about her capacity to match up with her own internal expectations, and those of other people, that she should be a perfect mother, who always understood and made allowances for every kind of behaviour.

The patients whose feelings and behaviour result in the kinds of upset I have just outlined are not 'mental' in the traditional sense. Stanton and Schwartz (1954) have described such phenomena in a mental hospital setting, but similar disturbances can very easily occur in a modified way in other situations.

We struggled with this approach for two or three years until it became plain that this kind of nursing would get us nowhere. So we began an investigation to try to understand what was really happening in the doctor–nurse–patient relationship.

5 · *The Ailment*

BY T. F. MAIN

When a patient gets better it is a most reassuring event for his doctor or nurse. The nature of this reassurance could be examined at different levels, beginning with that of personal potency and ending, perhaps, with that of the creative as against the primitive sadistic wishes of the therapist; but without any such survey it might be granted that cured patients do great service to their therapists and nurses.

The best kind of patient for this purpose is one who, from great suffering and from being in danger of losing his life or sanity, responds quickly to a treatment that interests his doctor, and thereafter remains completely well; but those who recover only slowly or incompletely are less satisfying. Only the most mature of therapists are able to encounter frustration of their hopes without some ambivalence towards the patient, and with patients who do not get better, or who even get worse in spite of long devoted care, major strain may arise. Those who attend the patient are then pleased neither with him nor with themselves and the quality of their concern for him alters accordingly, with consequences that can be severe for both patient and attendants.

We know that doctors and nurses undertake the work of alleviating suffering because of deep personal reasons, and that the practice of medicine, like every human activity, has abiding, unconscious determinants. We also know that if human needs are not satisfied they tend to become more passionate, to be reinforced by aggression and then to deteriorate in maturity, with sadism invading the situation, together with its concomitants of anxiety, guilt, depression, and compulsive reparative wishes, until ultimate despair can ensue. We need not be surprised if hopeless human suffering tends to create in ardent therapists something of the same gamut of feeling.

It is true that he who is concerned only with research and is less interested in therapeutic success than in making findings will not be frustrated by therapeutic failure; indeed, he may be elated at the opportunity for research it provides; but such workers are not the rule among therapists. In much of medicine it is not difficult to detect something of the reactions I have described, together with defences of varying usefulness against them. An omnipotent scorn of illness and death, the treatment of patients as instances of disease, the denial of feeling about prognosis, are devices some doctors use to reach at something of the detachment of a research worker, which permit them to continue their work without too painful personal distress about the frustration of their therapeutic wishes. Refusal to accept therapeutic defeat can, however, lead to therapeutic mania, to subjecting the patient to what is significantly called 'heroic surgical attack', to a frenzy of treatments each carrying more danger for the patient than the last, often involving him in varying degrees of unconsciousness, near-death, pain, anxiety, mutilation, or poisoning. Perhaps many of the desperate treatments in medicine can be justified by expediency, but history has an awkward habit of judging some as fashions, more helpful to the *amour propre* of the therapist than to the patient. The sufferer who frustrates a keen therapist by failing to improve is always in danger of meeting primitive human behaviour disguised as treatment.

I can give one minor instance of this. For a time I studied the use of sedatives in hospital practice, and discussed with nurses the events that led up to each act of sedation. It ultimately became clear to me and to them that, no matter what the rationale was, a nurse would give a sedative only at the moment when she had reached the limit of her human resources and was no longer able to stand the patient's problems without anxiety, impatience, guilt, anger, or despair. A sedative would now alter the situation and produce for her a patient who, if not dead, was at least quiet and inclined to lie down, and who would cease to worry her for the time being. (It was always the patient and never the nurse who took the sedative.)

After studying these matters the nurses recognized that, in spite of professional ideals, ordinary human feelings are inevitable, and they allowed themselves freedom to acknowledge not only their positive but also their negative feelings, which had hitherto been hidden behind pharmacological traffic. They continued to have permission to give sedatives on their own initiative, but they became more sincere in tolerating their own feelings and in handling patients, and the use of sedatives slowly dropped almost to zero. The patients, better understood and nursed, became calmer and asked for them less frequently.

This story is, of course, too good to be true, and I have to report that since then occasional waves of increased consumption of aspirin and vitamins have occurred. Such a wave seems to have little to do with patients' needs, for it occurs whenever a new nurse joins the staff or when the nursing staff are overworked or disturbed in their morale.

The use of treatments in the service of the therapist's unconscious is – it goes without saying – often superbly creative; and the noblest achievements of man in the miracle of modern scientific medicine have all been derived therefrom. It is deeply satisfying to all mankind that many ailments, once dangerous, mysterious, and worrying, offer the therapist of today wonderful opportunities for the exercise of his skill; but with recalcitrant distress, one might almost say recalcitrant patients, treatments tend, as ever, to become desperate and to be used increasingly in the service of hatred as well as love; to deaden, placate, and silence, as well as to vivify. In medical psychology the need for the therapist steadily to examine his motives has long been recognized as a necessary, if painful, safeguard against undue obtrusions from unconscious forces in treatment; but personal reviews are liable to imperfections – it has been well said that the trouble with self-analysis lies in the counter-transference. The help of another in the review of one's unconscious processes is a much better safeguard, but there can never be certain guarantee that the therapist facing great and resistant distress will be immune from using interpretations in the way in which nurses use sedatives – to soothe themselves when desperate, and to escape from their own distressing ailment of ambivalence and hatred. The temptation to conceal from ourselves and our patients increasing hatred behind frantic goodness is the greater the more worried we become. Perhaps we need to remind ourselves regularly that the word 'worried' has two meanings, and that if the patient worries us too savagely, friendly objectivity is difficult or impossible to maintain.

Where the arousal of primitive feelings within can be detected by the therapist, he may, of course, put it to good use, and seek to find what it is about the patient that disturbs him in this way. There is nothing new in categorizing human behaviour in terms of the impact upon oneself – men have always been able to describe each other with such terms as lovable, exhausting, competitive, seductive, domineering, submissive, etc., which derive from observation of subjective feelings; but the medical psychologist must go further. He must seek how and why and in what circumstances patients arouse specific responses in other human beings, including himself. If only to deepen our understanding of the nature of unconscious appeal and provocation in our patients, we need better subjective observations and more knowledge about the personal behaviour of therapists; and if such observations lead us also to the refinement of medical techniques, so much the better. To use an analogy: it is one sort of observation that some gynaecologists seem to have a need to perform hysterectomies on the merest excuse; it is another that some women seek hysterectomy on the merest excuse. It is not easy to say about a needless hysterectomy which of these is the victim of the other's wishes, which has the more significant ailment, and which derives more comfort from the treatment. In a human relationship the study of one person, no matter which one, is likely to throw light on the behaviour of the other.

In the light of these considerations I propose to discuss some events in the hospital treatment of a dozen patients. All were severely ill and before admission had received treatment at the hands of experts; some had already been in several hospitals and had received many treatments. Further treatment likewise did little to help them; for none was really well upon discharge from hospital and most were worse. The diagnoses vary from severe hysteria and compulsive obsessional state to depressive and schizoid character disorder. The patients were admitted at different times over a period of two and a half years, but I came to group them as a class of distinct feature because of what happened. The last of these patients was discharged over five years ago [before 1952], but I am still ashamed to say that I was pushed into recognizing common features by nursing staff who compelled me to take notice of events that had been for long under my nose.

It began this way. The nurses were concerned about a number of their members who had been under obvious strain at their work, and sought to know if this could be avoided. It was a question relating not to unstable women whose distress could have been regarded merely as personal breakdowns unconnected with work, but rather to valuable colleagues of some sophistication and maturity. The senior nurses met with me to discuss this matter, and I found that they were aware of several episodes of severe individual strain, almost of breakdown, that had occurred over the past three years. I had known of two breakdowns of clinical severity, but I was not aware of the others, which had been concealed by the individuals in question. These were now discussed in the open and every case was found to have been associated with the nursing of some particularly difficult patient who had not improved with treatment, and who had been discharged not improved or worse. These patients had been the subject of much discussion during and after their treatment, but even with the passage of time the nurse concerned had been unable to reach a workaday acceptance of the bad prognosis and the failure of treatment. We now found that in spite of having made intensive and praiseworthy efforts with these patients, far in excess of ordinary duty, at least one nurse – sometimes more – felt that she had failed as a person, and that if only she had tried harder, or known more, or been more sensitive, the failure would not have occurred. This feeling ran side by side with another – a resentful desire to blame somebody else, doctor, colleague, or relative, for the failure. Each nurse who felt thus was regarded with sympathy and concern by her colleagues as having been associated with patients who were dangerous to the mental peace of their attendants.

It was decided to meet twice a week as a group and to make a retrospective study of all cases that the group listed as major nursing failures. The list contained the dozen names of the patients I mentioned earlier. At that time none of us knew that we were setting out on a trail that was to take us months of painful endeavour to follow.

THE RESEARCH METHOD

At first it was difficult to discuss these patients except by resort to the rather lifeless terms of illness, symptoms, and psychopathology, medical and nursing procedures and intentions, and we made little headway. We had yet to discover the potency of group discussion as an instrument of research into relationships with patients. Slowly, following clues in the discussion, the group turned its attention to matters of private feeling as well as professional behaviour with these patients, but this was not easy, especially at first, and many times the group ran into difficulties revealed by silences, depressed inactivity, frightened off-target discussions, and distaste for the investigation by one or more of its members. Sometimes I was able to interpret the difficulty, but the other members did so as often. The group was tolerant of the difficulties of its constituent members, and was ready to slow up and wait for anyone who had found the development too fast or the going too heavy, but it stuck to its task and grew the courage step by step to reveal a surprising pattern of old unsettled interpersonal scores hitherto unrecognized by all of us, which had revolved around the nursing of these patients. Private ambitions, omnipotent therapeutic wishes, guilts, angers, envies, resentments, unspoken blamings, alliances and revenges, moves towards and against other nurses, doctors, and patients' relatives, were shown now both to have animated some of the nursing procedures offered these patients, and to have been concealed behind them. We had known that these patients had distressed the nurses, and had called forth special effort by them, but we were astonished to find out how much this was so, and how much feeling and complex social interaction had lain behind the events of patient management.

All the patients had been in hospital for several months and we turned next to study the records of their daily behaviour. From discussion of these the group was able to reconstruct and relive in detail, with more or less pain, the covert configuration of emotions within which these patients had been nursed. We were all aware that the therapeutic passions and intrigues which the group now proceeded to examine with frankness, and more or less pain, were matters of the past, but there was solid agreement – in which I share – that they could not have been examined *in vivo* and that the truth about them could be admitted to common awareness only after time had allowed feelings to cool and wounds had been licked. We were also agreed that only a group could achieve the capacity to recall past events with the merciless honesty for detail and corrections of evasions and distortions that this one required from and tolerated in its members. With each patient discussed, the nurses gave courage to each other and growing insights were used more freely, so that with later cases it was easier for the nurses to recognize and describe the quality of the patients' distress and their own emotional and behavioural responses to it. Finer observations were sometimes made about the later cases, and, when this was so, the earlier cases were rescrutinized for the presence or absence of corresponding phenomena.

All findings about any event had to be unanimously agreed by those involved before they were recorded. This led to difficulties when the behaviour of doctors came under discussion, for the group contained none. We now determined to invite the doctor concerned with the case when it was under discussion, but this was not a success. The group was now a year old and had grown an unusual capacity for requiring the truth without reserve, and a frankness about emotional involvement with patients, together with a number of sophisticated concepts which presented difficulties for anyone who had not shared in the development of the group's work. Moreover, the group was anxious to get on and was no longer as tactful about personal reticence as it had been when it began. One doctor refused the group's invitation. Two came once, but one declared afterwards that his job was with the patient's psychopathology and not with staff behaviour. (He borrowed the group's findings on one of his patients a year later and lost them.) A fourth came twice and was manfully helpful about his own involvement but was much upset by painful revelations. It must be remembered that these patients were not only nursing, but also medical failures, and, as I hope to show, had a remarkable capacity to distress those who looked after them.

The doctors were very willing to discuss their patients in terms of psychopathology and of treatment needed and given, but were uneasy when it came to matters of personal feeling. They could not discuss the details of their own difficult personal relationships with these patients, even in obvious instances of which the group was now well aware, except defensively, in terms of self-justification or self-blame. The group members were prepared for the doctors to have the same difficulties in discussing old staff mistrusts and covert manoeuvres over patients as they had experienced themselves, and were sympathetic when these proved too great to allow quick collaboration. The nurses already knew much about the doctors' behaviour with all of these patients, and, while critical, they were also charitable about it because it had been so similar to their own. It was clear to all how hard the doctors had tried with their patients, how they had worried, as had the nurses, had stifled their disappointments, and made further efforts, and how they, too, had worn themselves to their limit. It was soon clear that it was unfair to expect them to contribute freely about these matters, for they had had no opportunity of developing in the group, of sharing in its members' growth from reticence to frankness, in their pain of overcoming resistances, and in their pleasure at finding new ways of viewing their own behaviour. As one nurse said: 'You have to go through it yourself before you can feel easy about what we have found.'

The doctors' views outside the seminar were that these difficult patients needed better diagnosis, better interpretation of ever more primitive feelings, more precise understanding. They, too, were inclined to feel very responsible for the failure of treatment, to search for defects in themselves, and to hint at blame of others in the environment – nurses, doctors, or relatives.

Now these attitudes were exactly those with which the nurses had begun. The research group had to decide whether to put the brake on its own adventures and wait for the doctors to catch up in sophistication, or to continue without them, with all the deficiencies of information this would mean. The doctors, forewarned of difficulties and of criticism, and lacking the same group need as the nurses to investigate occupational hazards, had also carried more responsibility and were certain to experience prestige problems in the group. These matters would plainly make for heavy going and, I felt, would complicate an already difficult enough group task. Anyhow, I decided to proceed without their contributions and this account is the poorer thereby. The doctors' troubles with these patients are, however, known in general outline, and at least some features of their behaviour were made plainer.

We proceeded with our survey of hospital events in detail and then we came to the question of how far the patients' behaviour had been characteristic not of them but rather of the hospital setting. We therefore surveyed the responses evoked by them in others prior to admission and we made an interesting finding. In hospital, because they had received all sorts of unusual attentions, we had come to refer to them in the group as 'the special patients'. Now we found that they had been 'special' in the eyes of other people before they had come into hospital.

Before I leave the description of the group as a research instrument, using group discussion and scrutiny of records as its method, I must point out one clear gain. The nurses had owned painful distresses, concealed ailments connected with certain patients' ailments, and, by disclosing these in respect of themselves and each other, they arrived not only at an increased capacity to recognize insincerities in their daily work, but at personal easement in it. They became less afraid of difficult situations and surer at their craft.

MODE OF ADMISSION

Prior to admission these patients had evoked in their attendants something more than the exercise of practised skills. The referring doctors were level-headed people, some of ripe judgement and deserved reputation, but each felt his patient to be no ordinary person and each asked that she should be given special status and urgent special care. They made special appeals, and in their concern and distress were not content that their patients should be scrutinized and admitted by the ordinary procedures of the hospital. They made almost passionate demands for the waiving of routines because of the patients' distress, and they stressed the special helplessness and vulnerability of the patients in the face of stupid judgements.

The fact that some of these patients had been in mental hospitals and that several had a history of self-destructive acts in the past was mentioned – if at all – not as of warning significance but as an example of former wholly unsuitable handling. In two cases there was a clear statement that if the patient was not admitted soon, she would have to go to a mental hospital, the implication being that this disastrous step would be all our fault. Great stress was laid on the innate potential of the patient and the pathetic and interesting nature of her illness. Poor prognostic features were concealed or distorted and the group learned to recognize the phrases 'Well worth while' and 'Not really psychotic' as having been ominous special pleas. Personal relationships and past obligations between referrer and hospital doctor were traded upon where present, and four of these cases were first mentioned at friendly social gatherings after the hospital doctor had been offered drinks and a meal by the referrer. In every case the referrer also spoke to the hospital several times by telephone and sent one or more letters.

The referrers had all decided that their patient needed intensive psychotherapy and wished to leave little choice of decision to the hospital. Some seemed to fear that nobody but themselves could really get the hang of the subtleties of feeling in their patient, and that she would be in danger of being judged insensitively as unmanageable rather than 'special'. Some referrers asked for assurances that she would be handled with extreme care or by a particular doctor.

In all cases the referrer felt the patient to have been mishandled in the past by other doctors, institutes, or relatives, who had been unimaginative or unfeeling, limited in sensitivity, crude rather than culpable; and in some there was implied doubt that the hospital staff would have the same limitations.

Many people, doctors, friends, relatives, hospitals, and other agencies, had helped in the past, in their own ways, but few were on sincere speaking terms with one another. Most had been impressed with how little real understanding the others had shown and had tried to rescue the patient by giving lengthy unusual services; but all, in turn, had sooner or later felt that their aspirations were beyond their capacities and had sought somebody better than they, and had begged him to help. As can be imagined, the group called this 'the buck-passing phenomenon', but it was clear that when anyone had handed the patient on he had done so in apologetic distress, insisting to the patient on his goodwill and that this was for the best, but making it clear that for reasons beyond his control, and for which he was not to be blamed, he could do no more. All had felt keenly for the patient, and once she was admitted several of the prime helpers wrote letters or visited on her behalf; and letters to them from the patient led them to write to the staff in advisory, pleading, or admonitory ways. It was plainly difficult for them to relinquish to others full responsibility for the patient. The research group later came to the half-serious conclusion that whenever the correspondence file of a patient weighed more than 2 lb the prognosis was grave.

Our referring doctors were the most recent link in this chain of helpers. They, too, had failed to rescue the patient, were uneasy at their failure, and were inclined to blame others, especially relatives, but sometimes colleagues. They were clearly worried by the patient's distress, and wanted to rid themselves of their responsibility, with professions of goodwill. Concern for the patient was emphasized; impatience or hatred never. They asked for help for the patient of the kind they had devised, and wished to leave so little choice to us that it seemed as if we had to be their omnipotent executive organ. It was clear that whatever admission to hospital might do for the patient, it would also do much for them.

In some cases the patient belonged to more than one doctor at once, having gone from one to another without being, or wishing to be, fully relinquished by the first; but there was little consultation between these doctors, and entry into hospital was then less an agreed policy between all doctors and relatives than a determined act by the referrer wishing to rescue the patient from a situation and from people he secretly mistrusted.

All these patients were female. This gives no surprise in a hospital where two-thirds of the patients have always been female, but it may have other significance. Eight were either doctors, or doctors' wives, daughters, or nieces, or were nurses; a ninth had given blood for transfusion and then because of sepsis had had her arm amputated, with great uneasiness among the surgeons concerned. These medical connections are not typical of the usual hospital admissions, and raise the interesting possibility that these were patients who sought intense relationships with therapists because of their personal past (all of us have heard the story of the doctor's son who said that when he grew up he was going to be a patient). At all events, the referring doctor's freedom of decision was made more complicated by such a medical background, and his prestige in his local medical world was sometimes at stake.

IN HOSPITAL

I shall not describe the patients' personal histories, complaints, symptoms, moods, personal habits, nor the classical diagnostic features of their various states. These were of a kind commonly found in mixed psychiatric practice with severely ill patients, and none explains the nature of the object relations, nor why they, more than other patients with similar diagnoses, became 'special' and invoked in their attendants so much omnipotence and distress, so great a desire to help, and so much guilt at the gloomy prognosis.

Rather, I shall describe something of their behaviour and of the behaviour of the staff.

The last of these patients was discharged over five years ago and all the staff concerned have learned a lot since then, but it would be a mistake to suppose that these patients were in the hands of beginners, either in psychotherapy or in nursing. Of the seven doctors involved, at least three would be regarded as experts, two as well trained, and the others as serious apprentices. The nurses were all qualified but fairly young, and, like the doctors, keen to do good work. None of the staff – this may be a severe criticism – was of a kind that would easily admit defeat.

Each of these patients became 'special' after entering the hospital, some almost at once, others after a month or two. This was not only because of the referring doctors' wishes, their histories of ill-treatment by others, their difficult lives, or their medical relatives, but because of something in themselves. Not all severely ill patients are appealing; indeed, some are irritating; but all of these aroused, in the staff, wishes to help of an unusual order, so that the medical decision to treat the patient in spite of manifestly poor prognosis was rapidly made. The usual open assessment at staff conference tended to be quietly evaded, made indecisive, or regarded as unnecessary; or it was avoided by classifying the treatment as a special experiment. Each patient was felt to be a worthwhile person, who had been neglected, who could not be refused, and who, with special sensitive effort by all, should be given whatever chance there was without any red-tape nonsense. To every occasion one or other of the nursing staff also rose above her best, wishing to make a special effort to help, to rise above 'mere' routines, and to be associated with a compelling case in spite of the extra work it would seem to involve.

It is interesting that under special arrangements all of these patients fairly quickly acquired special nurses, usually one, occasionally two. Thereafter, this nurse engaged upon a relationship with the patient that became closer than usual, and both, because of the sharing of crises, became closely in touch with the therapist outside of the usual treatment sessions or case conferences. These nurses were regarded by the doctors and the patients and themselves as having a special feel for the patients' difficulties and a quality of goodness and sensitivity that was all-important.

The group came to call these features the 'sentimental appeal' (from the patient) and the 'arousal of omnipotence' (in the nurse). The nurse thereafter soon came to feel that she possessed a quality that the others lacked, and began to protect the patient from unwelcome hospital routines and unwanted visitors or staff. She would instruct other staff how they should behave towards the patient and directly or by scheming would ensure that the patient's need for special privileges or freedom was granted without much demur. She would modify or evade hospital procedures if these were distasteful or upsetting for the patient and be much more permissive and tolerant of special demands than was her usual custom.

The patient's need for special attention was, however, never satisfied except for the shortest periods, so that the nurse was led to demand ever more of herself. She came to feel that distress in the patient was a reproach to the insufficiency of her own efforts, so that the handling of her patient became dictated less by her decisions and more by the patient's behaviour. Most of these nurses believed, and were supported by the patient's doctor in their belief, that their efforts for the patient were of great significance, and that, by being permissive, even at heavy cost to themselves, they were fulfilling unusual but vital needs in the patient. The nurse usually felt that where others had failed the patient in the past by insensitive criticism, she, by her devotion and attention to the childlike wishes of her patient, could sufficiently still turbulent distress, so that the doctor could better do his work of interpretation.

As week after week went by the patients became more disturbed, but this was seen only as evidence of how ill they always had been basically, and of how much more devotion they needed than had at first been imagined. The nurse would remain with her patient during panic, anger, depression, or insomnia, soothe her with sedatives, in increasing amounts, protect her from unwelcome situations or unwanted stimuli, ensure that she had special food and accommodation, and special bedtimes, and was given attention immediately she needed it. More time, more sessions, more drugs, more attention, more tact, more devotion, more capacity to stand subtle demand, abuse, ingratitude, insults, and spoken or silent reproach were required of the nurse by the patient and by the 'in-group' around her, doctors and colleagues. The patient's wishes, covert rather than overt, were felt to be imperious in that they should stand no delay. Crises occurred of anxiety, depression, aggression, self-destructiveness. The nurse might have on her hands a patient sleepless, importuning, and commanding attention, distressed if the nurse wanted to go to the toilet or for a meal, liable to wander cold in her nightdress, perhaps ready to burn herself with cigarettes, bang her head against the wall, cut herself with glass, or dash outside. The nurse's time and attention became ever more focused on the patient so that she would voluntarily spend part of her off-duty, if necessary, with the patient.

The favourite nurse came to believe, from subtle remarks by the patient, that the other nurses, good and effortful though they were, did not have the same deep understanding, so that she would become the patient's unspoken agent, ready to scheme against and control colleagues whose behaviour she felt, through no fault of their own, to be unsuitable for her patient. Increasingly the nurse concerned found herself irresistibly needed by the patient, and sometimes by the therapist, to take over more and more responsibility for some of the patient's ego activities, to think for and decide for the patient, to see that she remembered her appointments with her doctor, to fetch and carry, to protect from stimuli, to supervise ordinary bodily functions, such as eating and bathing and lavatory activities. The nurse felt it was woe betide her if she did this badly or forgetfully. To a greater or lesser degree each of these patients ceased to be responsible for some aspect of herself, and with the most severe cases the nurse was expected to diagnose and anticipate the patient's wishes without the patient being put to the trouble of expressing them, to have no other interest than the patient, and to be sorry if she failed in this.

There was a queenly quality about some of these patients in the sense that it became for one nurse or other an honour to be allowed to attend them in these exacting ways, and by subtle means the patients were able to imply that unless the nurse did well, favour would be withdrawn, and she would be classed among those others in the world, relatives, previous attendants, etc., who had proved to be untrustworthy and fickle in the past. So skilled were these implications that some nurses became rivals to look after these patients, and felt it as a sign of their own superior sensitivity when the patient finally preferred them to another.

The disappointed, unfavoured nurse might feel shame, envy, resentment, and sulkily turn elsewhere for other comfort.

The patients were not merely insatiable for attentions such as conversations, interpretations, sedation, hand-holding, time, and other things that could be given purely as a matter of duty. They required that these attentions be given with the right attitude and even that the person giving them should do so willingly and with enjoyment. For instance, the nurse would be told, 'You are looking tired', in a tone that was less of concern than of reproach. Or she would be accused after making some considerable effort that she had not enjoyed doing it. Most of these patients were extremely sensitive to negative feelings in their human environment and the group called this 'paranoid sensitivity'. The nurse would, at a look of misery from the patient, feel guilty about any reluctance she might have had in providing something for her patient and feel afraid that the patient would detect this. For derelictions of duty or of feeling the nurse might feel punished by the patient's becoming turbulent or exposing herself to injury or threatening such a possibility. Nevertheless, there was something about the patients that made nursing them worth while.

Behaviour of the same order seems to have occurred with the therapists. Under the stress of treatment they gave unusual services, different from those given to other patients, more devotion, greater effort, with desperate attempts to be good and tolerant and to interpret the deeper meaning of each of the patient's needs, and to avoid being irritated or suppressive. They, too, felt their extreme worth for the patient. As the patients became more insatiable for attention, more deteriorated in behaviour, restless, sleepless, perhaps aggressive and self-destructive, and intolerant of frustration, the doctors' concern mounted and they were drawn increasingly – except in one case – into advising the nurses on management. The group came to recognize confusion of roles as typical of the situations that grew around and were created by the particular quality of distress in these patients. Therapists accustomed to non-directive roles would give advice on or become active in details of management. Nurses or doctors whose roles were of management only would become minor psychotherapists during crises, blurring their several roles and professional obligations. Once staff anxiety grew beyond a certain point, therapy became mixed with management, to the detriment of both. The therapist might advise nurses or encourage them to make further efforts, tell them to allow more sedatives if the patient could not sleep, to avoid frustrating the patient in various ways, to carry on sensitively and devotedly and to remain tolerant and friendly. Nurses whom the patient did not like came to be ignored by the therapist and he might try to get the more responsive kind. The nurse thus honoured would be resented by the others who felt hurt by the implications that they were too insensitive.

All of these patients had extra treatment sessions over and above the agreed programme, and for some there grew up an arrangement that, if the patient were badly distressed in the evening, she or the nurse could telephone the doctor and he would come to the hospital and settle the crisis by giving a session in the patient's bedroom. Increasingly, the therapist accepted his importance for the patient and, showing mistrust of the nurse's abilities to manage the patient well, began to take more decisions himself. Having been indulgent with sedatives, some nurses, alarmed at the dosage now required, would attempt to get the patients to accept less, but by distressing the doctor, sometimes by telephone, these patients would usually succeed in getting the nurses' decision reversed, until massive doses might be required daily.

The doctors' unusual attentions were, of course, regarded by them as being unorthodox, and they were uneasy that, no matter what they did, their interpretative work did not make the situation better. They pursued their interpretative work ever more intensely and more desperately and continued to do what they could to meet the patient's need for a permissive environment that could tolerate the patient without frustrating her needs. Neurotic diagnoses tended to be altered to psychotic terms and all the illnesses came to be regarded as even more severe than had at first been thought.

Thus, during their stay in hospital, these patients became 'special', and particular individuals became worn out in the process of attending to their needs. The patients, appealing at first, and suffering obviously, slowly became insatiable, and every effort to help them failed. Nothing given to them was quite enough or good enough, and the staff felt pressed and uneasy that they could not help more. Now this was like the situation that existed prior to admission with the patient and the referring doctor. But for the hospital it was more difficult to pass the case on.

I must now mention some of the effects on the other staff, those not involved, whom I will call the 'out-group'. These were not principally concerned in the treatment of these patients, but from time to time cared for them in minor ways on occasions when some member of the 'in-group' was unable to do so. They could be regarded as those whom the patient had not honoured. At first, in open, polite ways they would disagree that the patient should be handled with special devotion, and sometimes they doubted whether the patient should be handled at all except in a mental hospital. The in-group regarded this view as unworthy (although they did not say so openly), and the out-group thereafter concealed their opinion and felt unworthy or resentful or even envious of the verve and courage of the in-group. Later, as the patient became worse, the out-group would become bolder and would discuss among themselves their beliefs that the treatment of this patient was unhealthy, unrealistic, and a waste of time, and later still they would endeavour to keep out of what they felt scornfully, but secretly, to be a dangerous and unprofitable situation. They would resent the disturbance the 'special' patient created for them and their own patients, and then became increasingly critical among themselves of the in-group, blaming it for the patient's distress and criticizing its handling of the situation as being morbidly indulgent. Stanton and Schwartz (1949 a, b, c; 1954) have well described the subsequent fate of the in-group. Under the felt, but undiscussed, criticisms it is driven to justify its performance; it withdraws increasingly from contact with the out-group and concentrates on attending the patient, who, however, only becomes more distressed. Two languages now grow up, one describing the patient as 'getting away with it', 'playing up the staff', 'hysterically demanding'; the other using terms like 'overwhelmed with psychotic anxieties', 'showing the true illness she has hidden all her life', 'seriously ill'. The out-group now regards the in-group as collusive, unrealistic, over-indulgent, whereas the in-group describes the out-group as suppressive, insensitive to the strains on an immature ego, lacking in proper feelings. Our research group confirms that this was the case with these patients. The later development of the group situation was agreed to be as follows.

Eventually, the main nurse of the in-group, having lost the support of the out-group and the personal goodwill of colleagues once important to her, and needing but failing to get justification from her patient's improvement, would become too disturbed to carry on. She would become anxious, or ill, or would suddenly and unexpectedly become angry or in despair with the patient and now feel that it was fruitless to work with such an unrewarding patient or to do good work amid such colleagues. She might say that the patient was far too ill to be nursed outside a mental hospital or might develop the opinion that the patient should be given continuous narcosis or ECT, or be considered for a leucotomy. With the growth of unspoken disagreement between the in-group and the out-group these patients – who could sense unspoken tensions unacknowledged by the staff – would get worse and increasingly seek evidence of the reliability and toleration of the in-group and of its capacity to control the out-group. Then later, when the distress in the in-group mounted, the patients would become panicky, aggressive, and self-damaging, demanding and despairing or confused.

The therapist, the centre of the in-group, might now, in an effort to preserve his benevolence, advocate the least savage of the physical treatments mentioned, but he might consider others; he might say that he himself was prepared to carry on but felt that the other staff were incapable of giving more, or that because of the risk of suicide the patient should be sent to a closed hospital.

During their stay seven patients were, in fact, given continuous narcosis and one had a few ECTs. Four were discharged to closed hospitals, two dying there a year or two after admission from somatic illnesses to which they offered little resistance, one having had a leucotomy. One patient was discharged to an observation ward. One committed suicide in the hospital, and another did so after discharge to relatives who refused advice to send her to a mental hospital. Of five patients discharged home, one later had a leucotomy, three remained in analysis and are now leading more stable lives, and the other needed no further treatment.

Even when drawn from three hundred patients, such severe failures are dismal. It is true that the previous therapies of these patients – one had been in fifteen hospitals – had failed and that they were all referred as major problems, except one who was thought of as a straightforward neurotic; but failure, after so much effort, is bound to disappoint. These failures did more than disappoint – they left all concerned with mixed feelings of uneasiness, personal blame, and defensive blaming of others. They got under the skin and hurt.

Our findings agree with those of Stanton and Schwartz that certain patients, by having unusual but not generally accepted needs, cause splits in attitudes of the staff, and that these splits, if covert and unresolved, cause the greatest distress to the patients, who could be described as 'torn apart' by them. These two writers warn against easy assumptions that the patient is trying to drive a wedge between staff members, and they point out that the patient's distress can be dramatically resolved if the disagreeing staffs can meet, disclose and discuss their hidden disagreements, and reach genuine consensus about how the patient could be handled in any particular matter. We found, however, that the staff splits, while precipitated by disagreements over present events, occurred along lines of feeling and allegiances that had existed prior to the patient coming into hospital. These have too lengthy a history to be described here, but they were complex and hidden from us, until our painful study, under the mask of co-operative feeling by which every community defends itself from disruption. In other words, something about these patients widened and deepened incipient staff splits that would otherwise have been tolerable and more or less unnoticed. Some of the phenomena I have described, particularly the terminal social phenomena, are good examples of the social processes to which Stanton and Schwartz have drawn attention. Their research was not, however, able to include the part played by patients in situations of covert staff disagreement, or the nature of the patients' wishes. Because of the particular research instrument I came to use – group discussion – I am in a slightly better position to demonstrate the patients' part in increasing incipient disunity. I quote two examples.

One nurse told the research group that there was something about one patient that she alone knew. The patient had told it to her in confidence so that she had felt honoured and trusted more than any other nurse. She had respected the confidence and had spoken to no one about it. It was that the patient had once had a criminal abortion. The group listened to the nurse in silence, and then first one and then another nurse revealed that she, too, knew of this, had been told of it in confidence, had felt honoured, and had also felt that the others were too condemnatory to be told about it. We subsequently found that other patients had used similar confidences – which we came to call 'the precious little jewels of information' – to form special relationships with several nurses, making each feel more knowing than the others, and inhibiting them from communicating honestly with one another. It was as if the patient wanted each nurse for herself and that each nurse came to want the patient for herself. Thus, split and silenced, each was prepared to be sure that none of the others had the same inner awareness about what was good for the patient, and to feel that the others in their ignorance could only cause distress.

Here I am reminded of the way in which, prior to admission, various people had rescued these patients from others whom they mistrusted, and of how often the hospital's sensitivity in turn was mistrusted by the referrers.

My second example concerns a patient whom I visited because of a raised temperature, but whose psychotherapist was another doctor. She was emotionally distressed so I spent longer with her than I had intended and I emerged from my visit with the knowledge that I had a better feel for her emotional difficulties than her own therapist had. I realized in all fairness that this was not his fault; for I could not blame him for being less sensitive than I. I then spoke to the patient's nurse and saw from certain hesitations in her account that she believed that she had a better feeling for the patient than I had. Each of us believed the other to be lacking in feeling of the special sort needed. I spoke to her of my conjecture and found it to be correct, and we were able thereafter to find out that this patient had made more than ourselves believe that, while everybody was doing his or her best, all were really lacking in finer emotions, and only *one* person in the place was really deeply understanding – oneself.

DISCUSSION

I have had to condense and omit findings, such as the large number of minor somatic illnesses that these patients developed, the alarming capacity of at least one to venture, without discoverable physical cause, perilously near the edge of life, and the way in which, before and after admission, people tended to evade telling these patients the full truth if it were painful, but I have given the main outlines of some complex events which merit scrutiny.

I hope it is not difficult to see something of the nature of the distress suffered by the patients' attendants. These patients had an unusual capacity, quite different from that of other patients, to induce not only sympathetic concern but ultimately feelings of massive responsibility arising out of a sense of guilt, one might almost say guilt-by-association with an inconstant, untrustworthy, and harsh world. This staff guilt grew and, sooner or later, becoming intolerable, was dealt with by denial and by projection onto others, the harsh ones. In addition, denial of guilt was accompanied by compulsive reparative efforts and omnipotent attempts to be ideal. When these efforts failed to still the patient's reproachful distress, further guilt was experienced which, together with hatred, was further denied and projected, and further grand efforts were made at super-therapy. As a persecuting damaged object the patient received frantic benevolence and placating attentions until the controls of increased hatred and guilt in the staff became further threatened. Sedation and other treatments, physical and psychological, now came into use almost as coshes to quieten the damaged object that the patient represented. Manoeuvres and demands to get other staff to be kinder and more understanding also began. Finally, with the cover of staff goodwill cracking, the patient was transferred to other care, or treatment was abandoned, with everyone concerned feeling guilty but continuing to believe in the validity of his own viewpoint and openly or silently blaming the others.

It is to be remembered that these events were hidden and unremarked until searching study brought them to light, and I believe that similar study of difficult patients in other hospitals, outpatient clinics, private practice, and general practice would show similar hidden events. They can be discerned in the behaviour of those who attended these patients prior to admission to hospital, and though these patients are the most gross examples I can find, they are not unique. Whenever something goes wrong with certain distressed patients after lengthy and devoted care, it is not difficult to notice the kind of staff ailment I have described, the same blaming and contempt of others for their limitations of theory, ability, humanity, or realism, and the same disclaimers of responsibility. Many of you will be able to recall problems of managing severely distressed patients, and how often therapists find themselves covertly at odds with professional colleagues with whom they share responsibility, and how the patient goes from one to the other and from one crisis to another. When this happens it is rarely oneself who is wrong-headed, involved, or blameworthy, for one is simply doing what one knows to be in the patient's best interests. If, in the words of that convenient phrase, therapy has to be abandoned for external reasons beyond the therapist's control, we cannot help it. We simply did our best in the face of difficulties. With recalcitrant illnesses this end to a therapeutic relationship is far from unknown.

The question to which I now invite your attention is: What is it about such patients that makes for these difficulties? Perhaps there is no general answer, but I offer, with hesitation, some formulations from existing theory which may be relevant to the features I have described.

The suffering of these patients is noteworthy. Those who had not spent their lives for others as doctors or nurses were worth while for other reasons, and the majority could be roughly described as decompensated, creative masochists, who had suffered severely in the past. In her description of a patient whose torturing distress was similar to our patients', Brenman (1952) points out the use made by the masochist of the projection of his own sadistic demands on to others who are then cared for by self-sacrifice. Others have in somewhat different terms described similar phenomena (A. Freud, 1937; Klein, 1946). These patients, as their referring doctors said, were or had been or could be worth while, that is to say, they had shown some capacity for serving others at cost to themselves. But in none of these women had the defence of projection with masochism succeeded fully, and even before admission their suffering contained marked sadistic elements which were felt and recognized and resented more often by relatives than by doctors. Though they spoke of the world as being impossibly insensitive and demanding, these patients were themselves unremittingly demanding of love, and tortured others to give it by stimulating guilt in them, by self-depreciation and by the extortion of suffering. Self-neglect and helplessness cruelly reproached the world for being no good, and some of them seemed to wish to die in escape from an unproviding world. Tormented by childlike needs and rages, they tormented others also.

The angry response of the out-group and the readiness for

suffering of the in-group may be seen as sadistic and masochistic responses to the sado-masochism of these patients and their raging demands for nurturance, but this is not a complete view.

I am sure you will have noticed their need for material tokens of love and goodwill as well as the eventual insatiability, passion, and ruthlessness with which these were pursued. The hostility that reinforced these needs seems to have given rise to features that can be viewed in terms of Klein's work: fear of the tortured attendant as a retaliating object, appeasement of her by flattery and seduction, demands for more attention as reassurance against the possibility of retaliation. You will note also how these patients isolated and controlled the behaviour of their objects and counter-attacked by savage suffering and appeal when the revengeful potential of their damaged objects seemed great; and how they sought regular reassurance that the object and its goodwill were still alive, reliable, and unexhausted. These fruits of aggressive feelings are most easily discernible in the patient's relationship to the nurse, but there is no reason to think that the therapist enjoyed any immunity from them – indeed, the evidence is all to the contrary. The more the in-group insisted by its actions that it was not bad but good, the more the patient was beset with the problem of trusting it, and of needing proofs that it was not useless, unreliable, and impure in its motives. This in turn further stimulated the staff to deny hatred and to show further good, whereat the patient was beset with the return of her problems in larger size. Thus insatiability grew, and it is interesting to notice that every attention, being ultimately unsatisfying, had to be given in greater amount, poisoned as it was, not only by the patient's motives on the one hand, but by the in-group's hidden ambivalence on the other.

In spite of the fact that the patient frequently feared and attacked the in-group, she turned to its strength whenever she felt threatened by other agents. The attempts of the in-group to be all-powerful on her behalf may now be seen as a response to the patient's need to idealize it, and its belief in the badness of the out-group as its attempt to evade and deflect the patient's projection of sadism. Nevertheless, the in-group itself contained its own problems of mistrust, of finding good and bad among its own members. Mistrust of others made for such confusion in the roles of therapy and management that the nurse could be said to be inhabited not only by her own wishes, but by the wishes of therapists, which sometimes contrasted and warred within her. It is only a slight exaggeration to say that at times not only the patient but the nurse was confused about who was who.

Many of the severe panics, depressions, confusions, and aggressive outbursts of these patients may thus be viewed as deriving from the sadism that lay behind their suffering. But, while this explains the later aggressive secondary features, it does not explain the more naïve wishes that were noticeable, especially during the early stages of their therapeutic relations. These wishes were at that stage not aggressive or passionate, but seemed rather to concern an expectation in the patient that was difficult to meet. This simple basic expectation was that someone other than herself should be responsible for her; behind the aggressive use of suffering it was not difficult to see a basic discontent with life and its realities. This is found, of course, in all sick and suffering people. In the early stages following admission the nurses were not much tortured by the patient. In addition to all else they were moved by helpless, unspoken, and childlike qualities of appeals which became complex only later. The patient's aggressive use of distress can be viewed as sophisticated versions of the signals an infant uses to dominate his mother and bring her to help him. Like infants these patients had a simple, self-centred view of the world – it had to manage them because they could not manage it. Infants need an agent who, in the face of distress, ought to want to diagnose the need and the quality of the satisfaction sought, and the behaviour of our patients with their nurses seemed to contain such needs. The nurse had to undertake responsibility for many of the patients' ego activities which the patients seemed to wish to discard. Some would require her to behave as if she had no identity or biological independence of her own, but was rather a feeling extension of their own body.

The queenly honouring of the nurse with a task that she might regard as difficult is similar to the charming and friendly way in which a baby will deal with his mother. Anna Freud (1953) has pointed out that, like any parasite, the baby does not excuse his host for her failure but attacks her, reproaches her, and demands that she make up for her fault and thereafter be perfect. (I would add here that his queenly love comes first and his displeasure is secondary to imperfections in his host.) The mother is a part of the pair, taken for granted, without right to leave, and Anna

Freud has described the baby's sense of the personal loss of part of himself if his mother walks away. If the mother can give only one response (e.g. feeding) for all forms of distress, an addiction to this imperfect response is created for the assuagement of all needs, and this addiction can never be quite satisfying and therefore has to be given for ever. The situation can arise out of the mother's limitations, or anxiety, or stupidity, or from her pursuit of theories of child care. Perhaps any theory relentlessly applied creates an addiction.

These patients also fit the description of the early stages of infancy to which Winnicott has given the term pre-ruth. They needed more love than could easily be given and could give little in return except the honour of being cared for. They could be quieted but not satiated by desperate acts of goodwill, but they were afraid of the inconstancy of their object, so they would cling to what they had and seek more. The fact that they were aggressive towards and contemptuous of their objects need not blind us therefore to the fact that needing is an early form of love. But catering for the object's wishes is impossible in the early stages of development prior to what Klein calls the depressive position.

Balint (1952) points out that the infant requires his mother not only to be constant and to manage the world and his own body for him in automatic anticipation of his wishes, but also to enjoy it and to find her greatest joy in doing so, to experience pain when he is unhappy, to be at one with him in feeling, and to have no other wishes. He goes on to indicate that the impossibility of these requirements, except for the shortest periods, leads not only to a disconsolate, forlorn longing for this state, but to a fear of the impotent, helpless dependence on the object. Defences therefore arise against the state and its pain in the shape of denial of dependence, by omnipotence and by treating the object as a mere thing. The pain of not being efficiently loved by a needed object is thus defended against by independence; and under the inevitable frustration of omnipotence hatred of the object for not loving arises.

In these patients the need to be at one with the object could be seen in small ways, not, to be sure, in the angry, revengeful, or domineering behaviour, but in the occasional, early, moving helplessness, in the requests for small satisfactions, in the need for harmony in the relationship and for identity of purpose. The *later* guilt-driven obedience in their objects was very disturbing to the patients, but I am impressed with the nurses' enjoyment of the earlier simple tasks when both parties could be pleased, the one to give and the other to receive. The nurse truly enjoyed then the honour done her of being accepted by the patient. Smaller enjoyments of this sort also occurred when the patient's simple pleasure might consist of doing some small thing for the nurse. Perhaps it was the rapidly succeeding suspicion of the danger of being helpless and dependent in the future that led the patient to become independent, omnipotent, and demanding, and thus begin the cycle of guilt induction, omnipotent care from the nurse, insatiability, and suffering.

In drawing attention to these theories of infant behaviour I am in no way suggesting a common psychopathology for the various illnesses from which these patients suffered, which merit full study in their own right. Rather, the possibility arises that *certain* features of these patients, particularly those that give rise to common behaviour problems, may have primitive origins of a basic order. Nor do I suggest that proper nursing could cure these illnesses; only that the nursing response to these patients and the events of management are crucial moves in a primitive type of object relation that is strainful for all and, if not well managed, may become unbearable for all.

The splitting of the staff (including the splitting of the in-group) can be thought of as a wedge of the kind a child will drive between his parents, but, while this explanation will fit the aggressive splitting activities of the patient, it does not fit the fact that shortly after admission of a patient the nurses would compete with each other to respond to her silent appealingness. The patient was involved in the split from the first and was later active in maintaining it, but did not seem to cause it in the first place. I am reminded more of the rivalries formed among a group of middle-aged women when a baby whose mother is absent begins to cry, and of the subsequent contest among the women for the honour of being allowed to be of service to him, that is, to be actively distressed by the baby's distress and made actively joyful by his joy. In such an innocent way the baby may evoke rivalries that already existed within the group in a latent form. He may then become distressed by these rivalries and even make them worse in his search for security; but in the first place he may have wished neither to seek them nor to exploit them. It is true that our patients *later* became distressed, aggressive, and insatiable and then further divided their world in an attempt to control its imperfections, but they were also particularly sensitive and vulnerable to disharmony in those around them; and, as Stanton and Schwartz have shown, the resolution of felt but undeclared disharmony among their attendants can have a dramatic effect on patients' distress. I would suggest, therefore, that the earliest, but not the later, staff splits were caused by competitive responses in the staff to primitive but impossible appeals from the patient, and that the succeeding hidden competition among the staff led the patient to insecurity and then to the panics, mistrust, demand, hatred, and the later active sophisticated splitting activities I have described.

The patient's distress at the splits in the staff may be viewed in terms of the unhappiness experienced by a child whose parents are not on speaking terms and who is made happier by the restoration of a harmonious atmosphere in the home. But it might also be viewed in terms of an infant's distress when in the care of an ambivalent mother, or of a mother who misunderstands his needs and pursues, for her own reassurance, authoritative theories on child care. I am inclined to the latter possibility because the splits that distressed these patients contained no sexual preferences and because they were equally distressed when receiving ambivalent or determined but inappropriate care by one person, although I realize that this is not a conclusive argument.

The hopelessness, the omnipotent control of the object and the disregard for its purposes, may be seen as defences against the dependence of primitive love. Certainly the touchiness and the ruthlessness, as well as the growing insatiability and the mounting sadism that split the patient's mind and give rise to confusion, panics, depressions, and severe suffering, are inherent dangers with these patients. Lastly, I draw attention to the repetitive pattern of the traumatic rejections that beset these patients' lives, both before and after admission, and to the possibility that this contains compulsive elements.

SUMMARY AND CONCLUSION

I have described a behaviour syndrome in terms of object relations. Although gross forms are outlined, it is held that minor forms of it can be noted in most medical practice. The patients concerned bore various classic diagnoses, but constitute a type that cuts across the usual medical classifications and can be recognized essentially by the object relations formed. This syndrome is difficult to treat successfully, and tends to create massive problems of management. Further study is needed of its psychopathology, sociology, management, and treatment.

The patients suffer severely and have special needs which worry all around them. They tend to exact strained, insincere goodness from their doctors and nurses, which leads to further difficulties, to insatiability, to a repetitive pattern of eventually not being wanted, and to the trauma of betrayal; it also leads to splits in the social environment which are disastrous for the patient and the continuance of treatment.

Sincerity by all about what can and what cannot be given with goodwill offers a basis for management, although it leaves untouched the basic psychological problems, which need careful understanding, but it is the only way in which these patients can be provided with a reliable modicum of the kind of love they need, without which their lives are worthless. More cannot be given or forced from others without disaster for all. It is true that these patients can never have enough, but this is a problem for treatment and not for management.

It is important for such patients that those who are involved in their treatment and management are sincere with each other, in disagreement as well as agreement, that each confines himself to his own role, and that each respects and tolerates the others' limitations without resort to omnipotence or blame. It is especially important for each to avoid the temptation to induce others to become the executive instruments of his own feelings and wishes.

Believing that sincerity in management is a *sine qua non* for the treatment of the patients I have described, I offer one piece of advice. If at any time you are impelled to give advice to others (to be less hostile and more loving than they can truly be) – don't.

I cannot conclude without paying tribute to the nurses and doctors who allowed me to share the study of their difficult work, and without acknowledging the pleasure I have had in formulating with them these ideas.

6 · *Change of Approach*

BY DOREEN WEDDELL

Confusion of roles

Among many other things illuminated by the research group was the very great confusion of roles.

The nurse was imitating the doctor. In her long heart-to-heart talks with the patients the nurse inevitably felt that she must be therapeutic, that she must say the right thing. Since the doctor's knowledge of psychopathology helped him to do this, then she must know psychopathology – and her interest in it led her to read and learn about it in staff seminars. There was tremendous need to know what went on in the doctor's session with the patient, and to continue his work during the rest of the day. The nurse seemed at times to have no role of her own, though she had a great deal of knowledge which was disturbing rather than useful.

Meanwhile the doctor's role was also confused. He sometimes used the nurse as if she were a part of himself, a sort of minor doctor. He sometimes behaved as if he were the nurse, going to see the patient in the bedroom when the patient did not go to the consulting room, making drinks for the patient, even at times staying up at night with a particularly disturbed patient.

As the matron, I added to the confusion, for I had a direct personal relationship with the most ill patients and often felt that *I* was the one who knew what should be done, what the patient should be given and how he should be managed. And I would tell the doctor and the nurse what I thought. Then the nurse would not know whether to please me or the doctor when we disagreed.

To put it another way, the patient seemed to want a perfect parent, and all concerned with the patient felt impelled to be one.

At the same time, the situation was wide open to exploitation and some patients were adept at finding everyone's weak spot and arousing the strong emotions common in any triangular relationship.

The meaning of drugs

This confusion of roles was also reflected in the drug situation. We found that drugs and time were more or less interchangeable. Drugs were given when the patient was asking for time that the nurse could not give, or when she had already been with the patient for as long as she could stand. We found that the patient asked for drugs as a way of achieving extra nursing contact. Drugs were seen to be not just sedatives to gain an extra good night's sleep or occasionally to give relief from tension or pain. They were tokens of love, of being cared for – extra sweets at bedtime, so to speak. The drugs were known by their colour. The patient would say, 'I've tried the red one, sister, I'm tired of that, I'll have a yellow one tonight.' They seemed to the patient to be the little extra drops of heavenly potion that could be got if only he went about it the right way. And the nurse got caught up in the same idea and would think that an extra dose or a different drug would magically do the trick.

In general hospitals something of the same thing can happen with the patient who is in for a period of time, and for whom separation from his family is an especially disturbing experience, reactivating feelings and behaviour stemming from childhood situations. Time from the night nurse or night sister may be what the patient really requires. The sedative may be the token of being cared for and protected, an assurance of not being forgotten at the moment when the wish is for oblivion.

We changed this situation in two ways, through a redefinition of the roles and responsibilities of everyone in the hospital, and through certain administrative changes. The drug situation was sorted out as the roles of doctors and nurses became clearer.

We made a rule that drugs could no longer be given at the discretion of the nurse; they had to be definitely and directly ordered by a doctor, not just p.r.n. or s.o.s. This meant that whatever meaning the drug had to the particular patient would come more immediately into the psychotherapeutic session and be discussed there with the doctor. We recognized the *nurse's* need for drugs – not to take herself, but to give to the patient – because they were the only means whereby she could manage the situation. The question began to be asked: 'Who really needs the drug, the nurse, or the patient?' If it was the nurse, then how long could she last out and what could be done to help her? In time, this situation became so changed that a nurse could sometimes be heard to say, 'This patient will have to have a sedative, the doctor can't stand the racket!' But it is a friendly remark, in which the patient's part can be clearly seen.

Sedatives are no longer given as a routine. For those patients to whom drugs have a very special meaning, and with whom there is bound to be a fight, relationships such as those described can now be worked out with codeine or aspirin rather than with barbiturates. Sometimes vitamins are the coinage. Extra cups of tea or milk will often do just as well, and if the patient can get these for himself the opportunity for fight or frustration can often be further minimized.

It must be emphasized that the very real intra-psychic pain experienced by the patient is fully recognized with sympathy and understanding, but experience has shown that sedatives as such do not usually help the situation, particularly when given over a period of time.

REDEFINING ROLES

Initially, the redefinition of roles and responsibilities was undertaken by the medical director, the principal administrative officer, and myself. Then each of us discussed the situation in our own departments so that eventually every member of the staff of the hospital had considered and defined his or her own role in various working situations. The whole process took about two years.

To summarize briefly, the following questions were asked: Who is responsible to whom and for what? Who provides what service and for whom? Once these questions have been answered to everyone's satisfaction, rivalries, power-seeking, and abrogation of responsibility can be seen and understood, and consequently minimized in effect. Once the executive structure of the hospital organization is clearly defined, manipulations by patients and staff for their own ends can be seen for what they are. The situation is kept under constant review because each new staff member inevitably shapes his or her role according to his or her personality and capacities. This ensures that the structure is defined but not rigid.

Clinical roles

The discussions about clinical roles and responsibilities naturally centred on the patient. We began thinking about what happened to him when he came into hospital. During the period 1948–51 the most obvious occurrence had been regressive behaviour. To what extent were we responsible for this? Did we foster an expectation in the patient that he would be cared for, thought for, looked after? In acute illnesses things have to be done for the patient; usually he is already feeling and behaving more like a child than an adult; and the essence of skilful nursing is to sense and supply his need. With patients whose difficulties are mainly experienced as disturbances of relationships with other people, the nursing task is quite different. To what extent did we help the patient to maintain his contact with the real world – his family, work, and friends – even though these were the situations in which he experienced pain? In what situations did he experience greatest difficulty? How could we help him to face them?

Answering these questions helped us to redefine the nurse's role.

The role of the nurse

The staff began to see that their task was not so much to be all-giving, all-pleasing mothers, who would never frustrate their children, as to be ordinary human beings, walking alongside and working with their patients, not just looking after them. To think *for* the patient in every situation is right and proper in the nursing of acute illnesses, but even then only during the early stages of the illness. Once this is over the nurse's task changes and she has to help the patient to face the problems of returning to home and work. This is where nursing in a general hospital comes near to the nursing approach I am trying to describe.

The nurse began to see that her role was to be available when wanted, rather than to have to be used for reasons of her own satisfaction or prestige; that her task was to be interested not in the deep emotional problems of the patient, but in his actual difficulties of daily living – at home, at work, and at play. She found that in discussing practical ways of approaching and solving these problems with the patient, in putting her point of view on occasions, she had a task that was essentially nursing, though the relationship provided satisfactions of a different order from those experienced in traditional nursing. She could be a woman with many capacities and interests of her own; she did not have to be a pseudo-doctor or perfect mother. The patient could then be thought of not as a child but as an adult, a citizen, with diminished capacities perhaps, yet nevertheless a responsible person, who had something to contribute to, as well as expectations of, society.

This approach called for major changes in two areas of the nurse's own life. If she was to be interested in the patient's day-to-day work, home, family, difficulties, and pleasures, she needed to know something of the problems and feel something of the same life stresses and enjoyments herself. If she took responsibility for her own way of living she would know what it was like to manage on a tight budget for food, clean the house, count the cost of entertaining, spend time on ordinary chores. So a change took place in the nurse's actual living quarters and she began to take more responsibility for providing her own food, cleaning her own room, and managing her own daily life in the way in which most people have to. It was at this time that the traditional nurse's uniform was changed. Nursing staff now wear suits or dresses of one colour and design, suitable for ordinary social situations.

These changes, together with the development of a changed medical and administrative structure, led to new nursing skills and satisfactions.

ADMINISTRATIVE CHANGES

The administrative changes were mainly to enable the medical units of doctors, nurses, domestic staff, and patients, each with its own area of the hospital, to become more self-reliant: for example, to enable each unit to work out its own particular procedures, at the same time taking more responsibility for the daily household tasks that any family expects to do for itself, thus giving the patients a chance to move from invalidism to reasonably healthy living. Each medical unit now had a financial budget within which it could buy required items. Each unit became responsible for providing a certain service for the whole hospital, a focal area where the staff, nursing and domestic, could work together with patients.

PRACTICAL NURSING

The nurse now embarks on a needed practical task and meets and talks with patients in the course of it. This has changed the nurse–patient relationship from a mutually dependent one to a reciprocal and mutually supporting one of equality. Sometimes the patient can do a task much better than the nurse, or can show the nurse how to do something. This change from working *for* to working *with* patients is a different way of looking at nursing. On the one hand, it brings back within its scope tasks that have been eschewed as domestic and not thought of or undertaken by professional nurses. On the other, there is opportunity to learn new skills and a chance to understand the relationships that develop round the task between individuals, in the serving of food, the mending of linen, the choosing of furnishings and colour schemes, and so on. Thus new satisfactions are provided and nursing interests are considerably expanded. The nurse has become group- and community-minded. She is concerned with understanding the patient's relationships in various situations rather than his psychopathology. Applied to the convalescent wards of general hospitals this last sentence could read: 'She can become interested in the patient's relationships inside and outside the hospital as well as in his disease.'

The group care of patients that is undertaken in some hospitals gives similar opportunities for the nurse to know about the patient's family, his difficulties and pleasures at home or at work, his anxieties about returning home and meeting colleagues. The nurse may be able to suggest ways of helping the patient with these problems. She can ask herself: How can I help him while he is still in hospital? What services does the hospital provide, through various staff members, that patients or their friends could provide for themselves? How can relatives be helped to feel that the patient is a member of their family and not the property of the hospital? How can the patient be helped to remember that ultimately he is responsible to himself for himself?

In considering the twenty-three hours of the day that the patient is not with the doctor, we asked how the patient spent his time, and what sort of work could be expected of him inside or outside the hospital. We examined every work situation in the hospital and asked ourselves such questions as: Who is really responsible for this task? Who has the power to make or mar this situation? Who really feels the brunt of any decision about this? Can the patient be helped to help himself? What service does the hospital provide for the patient that the patient could provide for himself? How far is living in hospital similar to the kind of living the patient might achieve outside the hospital? What is the nursing task in relation to a particular situation? As a result we found that most patients could take quite a lot of responsibility for managing their own lives. There was no reason why *they* should not decide what time they would go to bed, what time they would get up, when they would have meals, what sort of meals they would have, how they could look after hospital property. If the task is defined within reasonable limits, it can be accomplished.

The same approach can be useful in wards where patients are becoming ambulant and on their way to discharge from hospital. How do they spend their time? What tasks would they enjoy doing if allowed to? What can they do together with their relatives and friends? How can patients be helped to take the initiative and feel responsible for themselves and what they do?

Night duty

We found that the reduced consumption of drugs and this new approach radically changed the night-time situation. In the early years we had at least three nurses on night duty. Now we have one sleeping in the hospital, and only an orderly actually up at night, whose task it is to call the nurse if anyone requires anything.

So long as we had nurses on duty we had patients up and about – they needed each other: the nurse needed someone to talk to in the lonely hours, the patient wanted to know what was going on; it was a mutually collusive situation. Nowadays it is quite rare for anything to happen after 11 p.m. When we first began this system the nurse stayed up until 1 a.m. and then went to bed, but we found the same phenomenon – patients stayed up too. Now the whole hospital is pretty well bedded down by 11 p.m. without any administrative action at all, just as a family sets its own night-time routine, and people go to bed when ready.

As a result of these various changes, many situations that had, in the past, given rise to disagreement and tension between patients and staff became, instead, opportunities for co-operation between the patients themselves and between patients and staff, in which the staff could sometimes help the patients to see what they were doing.

TRAINING THE NURSE

We ask that the nurse should be herself, responding to the patients as she would to anyone else, but we also ask that she be prepared to look at and try to understand what is happening between herself and the patient, between the patient and other members of the community. We ask that she be sensitive to and capable of talking about what she feels. If she feels angry about or particularly attracted to a patient, these are facts to be aware of, facts that one or other member of the therapeutic team can know. She is asked to try to discover why she felt as she did at that moment, what it was in the patient that provoked it in her, and if she has observed this particular characteristic of the patient in his relationship with other people. If the nurse can comprehend something of what has occurred, it may result in some alteration of her response to the same sort of stimulus on future occasions. She may find that she will begin to deal with a similar situation in a slightly different way.

This way of working is not taught dogmatically but is implicit in the general approach and in the kind of question that the nurse is asked during staff discussions. We ask that she should be sincere with the patient, that she should always be honest and not try to hide, hedge, or cover up. (The patient usually senses what is happening anyhow.) We ask that the nurse shall try to understand what is happening in the complex pattern of relationship between the patient and herself, and have sufficient inner freedom to learn and develop.

Teaching[1]

The main teaching is aimed at giving an understanding of human emotional development from infancy to old age, on the basis of 'Psychology Applied to Nursing' (Weddell, 1955). In this way it is possible to show the links between childhood development and later adult character formation. This is done through seminar and case discussion, giving the nurse plenty of opportunity to talk

[1] See also Chapter 3, and, for later developments in teaching, Chapter 20 – Ed.

about her working experiences and to relate theory with practice. No formal lectures are given; reading is encouraged, and there are frequent opportunities for discussing in groups what has been read. Children are admitted to the hospital with their mothers, but the nursing staff also go to a day nursery during part of their training so that when we talk about children it is linked with actual experiences, which are discussed with a view to understanding what is happening at a particular time.

In my experience, psychology can only be taught on the job, at the moment when something is happening, when the actual emotional impact of a situation is being felt. Formal teaching of theoretical psychology is of little use to the nurse or to the patient. When teaching takes place in the working situation, linked with case discussions and reading material, something that is warm and useful is made available to the nurse, and theory becomes alive.

One of our students put it very well. We had been discussing the rivalries of children aged two to five years, and how jealous they could be of their brothers and sisters and of other people coming into the family circle. The nurse told me that she had heard all this before and that she knew it was true in a kind of way and was quite prepared to accept it because so many people affirmed it. But until recently, secretly inside herself she had always felt that *she* had never really had any rivalry problems; her sister was so much older that this kind of thing had not happened to her in her life. The other day, however, when she was reading Susan Isaacs's book, *Social Development of Young Children* (1933), she came across the phrase 'and when strangers came into the house'. The word 'strangers' reminded her of an occasion when she was quite young, when a stranger came into her home bringing two younger children, and she remembered how upset and difficult she had been at the time. To use her own words: 'Suddenly a whole flood of memories returned, ideas and incidents I had forgotten. And I realized at that moment just how vivid the experience was and how these things can be forgotten.' She said it was a most revealing moment, which somehow made much more sense of all sorts of other things she had previously accepted only intellectually.

Another point is that satisfactory teaching can occur only at the pace at which the students themselves can accept it, and one must be in fairly close touch with the students in order to be able to meet this requirement.

At report-time nurses are encouraged to report not only what has happened to the patients but also what is happening to them, how they have coped with the day's experiences, what they said and did when they felt frustrated or angry or pleased.[1] Talking things over helps to increase understanding and to some extent makes the patient or the situation less of a burden. It seems to me that if the nurse can understand how the patient is feeling by experiencing within herself something of the patient's emotion, if she can put what she feels within herself into words either to the patient or to someone else, a satisfactory relationship is achieved or maintained. When the nurse does not understand, when she feels irritated or burdened, either she will go on chewing over the situation inside herself, with probably increasing tension, or she will get fed up, shrug her shoulders, and feel it's not worth bothering about. Alternatively, she may resort to blaming techniques – that the trouble is with the doctor or another nurse – and this sort of reaction may lead to some disturbance of her relationship with the patient or the doctor or other nursing staff. When she can discuss what has happened she can, so to speak, get the un-understood experience outside herself and, examining it with someone else, come to know more about what may have happened (Money-Kyrle, 1956).

Observation and communication

We put great stress on observation and communication, not only as methods of teaching, but also as nursing skills. Acute, sensitive, and accurate observation has always been the basis of the best nursing. In general hospitals, observation of acutely ill patients often leads to immediate action. With emotionally disturbed patients many facts may have to be observed, recorded, and understood over a period of time before any action takes place. Just as accurate observation of the subtleties of change in the acutely ill patient speeds the introduction of the required treatment, so accuracy in recording the subtleties of behaviour in an emotionally disturbed patient leads to a greater understanding of what may be occurring. In this kind of nursing the difficulty is how to communicate these subtleties, which are often more in feeling terms than in clear behaviour. This is why the nurse's own feelings about a patient are important. What the patient is evoking in the nurse

[1] For later developments in reporting, see Chapter 20 – Ed.

is a fact to be noted and understood in the total pattern of the patient's relationships with other people.

We have found that quite frequently a patient will tell one member of the nursing staff one particular small item of secret information that he says he does not want anyone else to know. He makes a special communication, which becomes a special bond between him and the nurse. Later, we found that very often the patient had told two or three other people the same thing, but none of them knew that the others had this precious bit of information and all of them were to some extent uneasy because of this thing which could not be communicated.[1] A mild version of this phenomenon occurs daily with people who cannot keep a secret but implore others to do so for them. We teach new nurses the significance of this kind of bargain made with a patient, so that they can exchange information with other nursing staff, though at the same time there is a professional ethic about communication with other than medical or nursing staff.

The nurse gains her first experiences in this hospital by being concerned with new patients. All new patients come for an assessment period, which provides her with a limited and well-defined task. She is asked to be aware of and to describe the kinds of relationship the patient develops in the hospital and with her as the nurse; the effect that coming into hospital is likely to have on the patient and on the family; what attractions there are for the patient outside the hospital; what are the patient's and the family's expectations from treatment; how easy or difficult it will be for the patient to leave hospital. A description of these matters is presented at the medical conference.

To summarize our approach to nursing: the nurse is interested in and concerned about all the patient's relationships inside and outside the hospital. She is concerned for the family with one of its members in hospital, she is interested in the patient's work inside or outside the hospital, she works with the patient on ordinary household chores. She does not consider the patient's feelings or behaviour as good or bad, right or wrong, but seeks to understand them, describe them, and perhaps help the patient to see what effect they are having on other people. Her skill and understanding are directed not only to the individual but to group situations, to

[1] See also Chapter 5.

the management of numbers of people, to the significance of leadership roles, and to phenomena such as scapegoating, isolation, and so on.

Although each nurse has a case-load of individual patients, much of her time is spent in a group situation and in the management of what could sometimes be called a somewhat difficult household. The satisfaction of her work lies in the practice of household arts, with opportunities for relationships with a wide variety of people and for the development of special skills in management. Teaching is done through discussion of what actually takes place: recalling who said and did what in a particular situation and discovering what other ways there might be of interpreting and handling such a situation.

7 · *Nursing New Patients as a Learning Situation*

BY HAZEL EDWARDS

Patients are referred to the Cassel Hospital by psychiatric departments attached to teaching hospitals, by consultant psychiatrists, and by general practitioners. Each medical unit in the hospital has its own waiting-list, and the consultant in charge sends for the patient when there is a vacancy. A brochure describing the hospital and the patients' activities is sent to the patient before his admission, and he will have heard something of the hospital from his referring doctor. To prepare for his admission, the senior sister of the medical unit arranges accommodation with the housing representative (a patient).[1] The other patients in the unit are told of his expected arrival. The nurse concerned with his admission reads his notes, and acquires some knowledge of his past difficulties.

ADMISSION PROCEDURE

The patient and his relatives are met by the nurse who will continue to be his nurse during the assessment period and afterwards, if he remains for treatment. He is taken to his medical unit and to his bedroom, and is introduced to his room-mates and any other patients met *en route*. He is shown round the hospital with his relatives. He sees the dining-room and the servery where later he will take his turn in serving and washing up; the workroom where he can do pottery or painting, and perhaps some minor maintenance jobs for the unit. He also sees the telephone box where personal calls may be received from or made to relatives or friends. He is shown the common rooms where he can watch television, listen to the radio, and meet other patients and friends;

[1] See Chapter 8 – Ed.

he may be asked to help with the daily cleaning of these rooms if they are in his unit area. He is introduced to the medical secretary, and makes practical and financial arrangements for his stay in hospital.

After the general tour of the hospital the patient can talk privately with the nurse. This begins a relationship of confidence, so that later he can come to see her when he wants to, knowing that she has sympathy with his problems and would like to help. His relatives are also given an opportunity to talk with the nurse.

During the assessment period, which lasts about a fortnight, it is the nurse's task primarily to be available to the patient, to make appointments for him with the psychiatrist, psychologist, and others, to present the hospital in such a way that it may be useful to him, and to help him to become aware of what he may be able to contribute. She will let him get on with the process of adapting to and using the community with as little intrusion as possible, being as observant as she can. She tries to understand the relationship the patient is making with her, how he uses her and how she feels about him, and how he pictures the hospital and treatment. He might have come expecting immediate relief of his symptoms, or perhaps he sees the hospital as yet another futile attempt to get him better. In observing the relationships he makes with the other patients she may become aware of how he feels about people and how they respond to him. She discusses the problems that will face the patient on discharge from hospital. Will his job be kept open for him? How will his family feel about his return? These things help to build up a picture of the patient as a member of a family, with particular difficulties at home, at work, and in social situations.

The nurse sees the patient's relatives in order to discover the attitudes and practical problems of his family. It may be that the family resents the patient's coming for treatment or, again, the patient may have sought treatment only in response to family pressure. Is he the breadwinner? If so, have arrangements been made for the support of the other members of the family? Do they expect the hospital to deal with this matter? Do they resent offers of help? The nurse's task is to try to understand the difficulties and to redirect inquiries, where appropriate, to local authorities, housing officers, employment bureaux, welfare officers, and so on. She has been in touch with these agencies in the past, and she can provide the link between the family's need and the resources available. The nurse may find the family a useful ally in her work with the patient. Certainly, her contact with the family will help her to a better understanding of the patient and his problems.

LEARNING AND TEACHING

When a new nurse comes to the hospital she accompanies a senior nurse in her work, and is with her when she admits a new patient. She hears what is said and notices as much as she can. Later, she and the senior nurse discuss the situation; this is where formal teaching begins. The trainee asks questions about the management of the patient, and comments on what she has observed. The senior nurse explains why she responded to the patient in the way she did, and perhaps mentions other ways of management. This exchange between teacher and student allows for the possibility of inappropriate responses to become apparent. It is sometimes reassuring for a trainee to realize that a nurse with more experience may make mistakes in management, yet is still able to discuss the matter critically and not as if it were a major tragedy. It is really by personal observation in a working situation and by free discussion afterwards that the nurse begins to understand her role with emotionally disturbed patients.

One of the difficulties in this work is communication of the nurse's observations in writing. How much can she say? What should be left out? How can she say the essential things in the best possible way with no words wasted? What seems significant to one person may not be so important to another.

For teaching purposes we find that the daily verbal report is a useful occasion for discussion; a daily record of basic facts is also kept, from which information is extracted for the nursing report at the assessment conference.

After being an observer for a time the trainee will work with patients on her own. The senior nurse will be available for discussion when the trainee has first admitted a patient, or if any behaviour difficulties occur during the day. Talking it over with someone not involved helps the trainee to clarify her ideas and feelings, and this, in turn, helps her to understand what she has observed.

In the formal teaching programme, the nurse has weekly

discussions with the matron on emotional development from infancy to old age. She also has discussions with a senior nurse on working with families. Another senior nurse meets with the trainees at regular intervals to help them to understand the present behaviour of patients in the light of what may have been the patients' past experiences. For instance: the trainee is working with a young married woman with two children; the woman is extremely anxious and frequently needs to see the nurse and know she is around, yet at the same time she is seldom really able to make use of her. The patient constantly asks questions and seeks advice, then disregards it. The problem is really one of disturbed early relationships causing insecurity and difficulty in trusting people; the patient has to make people useless in order to prove how badly she is being treated. These early difficulties of the patient are being reflected in her present inability to use the nurse, and in the way in which she makes it known that some other nurse is of more help to her.

Such a situation presents difficulties for the new trainee. Naturally she wishes to prove herself a 'good nurse' and feels her prestige threatened when the other nurse is always the chosen one. She may feel that if she gives a little more time and attention, or tries harder, she will be accepted by the patient. That this really won't help can be illustrated in the teaching situation as follows.

All trainees meet for discussion with the senior nurse. After some talking it may come out that one nurse is uneasy about the management of one of her patients. The senior nurse may then ask for an example of what is happening. The nurse may say that she always seems to find herself involved in argument of one kind or another with this patient. For instance, the patient has asked her doctor for some particular medicine and has understood that she could have it, but in fact this prescription has not been ordered. Or, if the right medicine has been prescribed, she wants it given in a different way or at a different time. If it is a medicine that has to be diluted, the patient has been given too much water or too little, or she insists on washing out the glass to make sure that she has the last drop. And frequently, after she has taken the medicine, the one she had before was much better anyway! This patient always seems to be wanting something, just half a minute after everyone else has finished, or just at the last minute before the nurse is going off duty, 'and when I have been available all the afternoon, or just when I'm going to a meal. She always seems to be discussing her problems with the evening duty sister, when I, her own nurse, have been on duty all day, and she could have come to me at any time.'

We find, during discussion, that this patient always says that another nurse is much more helpful than her own nurse and seems to understand her much better; in fact, is the only one who knows how she feels. The rejected nurse may go on to say that she has tried very hard to be particularly careful in her approach to this patient because she is aware of the patient's difficulties.

It is easy to see that, in such a situation, the favoured nurse may begin to think that there is something in what the patient keeps saying, that she really is better with the patient; and privately she begins to blame the rejected nurse for upsetting the patient by her inefficiency. Both nurses have the opportunity to talk about this with the senior nurse. They may then begin to understand how this patient has to go on repeating earlier relationships and difficulties. The rejected nurse can see that it is not necessarily she herself who is unacceptable. The patient is responding to her as if she were one of the people of her past experience, making the nurse feel angry, incompetent, and guilty, as other people have been made to feel before her.

At such a time it is possible to see how strong feelings are aroused, which belong (for both the nurse and the patient) to patterns of behaviour stemming from childhood days. When this is recognized, the nurse's confidence in herself is less threatened by the supposedly better nursing of her colleague. She can begin to look at methods of management which will help the patient to see what she is doing, how she sets one person against another, always prefers the nurse she cannot have, frustrates people, and makes them feel angry and guilty.

This illustrates one way in which a discussion group can be used for teaching purposes. The everyday work of the nurse is co-ordinated in a learning-teaching relationship, and in the teaching situation there is an attempt at understanding the subtleties of the nurse–patient relationship, which is the essential skill in nursing.

8 · *Patient Community Organization*

BY BLODWEN WIGLEY

Patients first started holding weekly meetings in 1946. They were conducted by their elected chairman and secretary, with staff help, and discussed hospital procedures and patients' welfare and activities. At that time the chairman and secretary had the right to take up with the appropriate staff any matters arising out of these meetings. The patients' meetings were also responsible for organizing recreation and entertainment. Subcommittees formed as occasion demanded.

One important committee dealt with what is known as 'housing'. The allocation of beds to patients has never been a simple matter in the Cassel Hospital, partly because of the layout of the building and partly because of the length of stay of patients. The accommodation consists of rooms containing from two to five beds, and a very few single rooms.

When the nursing staff decided where patients should sleep there were always complaints: 'Mrs So-and-So can't bear to stay in the room with Miss Such-and-Such another minute.' 'Mr So-and-So snores, no one can sleep in the room with him.' Often, more violent criticisms were made of the personal behaviour of some of the patients.

Sometimes the medical staff would try to arrange changes of room-mates. Sometimes the nursing staff could manage without too much difficulty. A situation developed in which a patient who made enough fuss or had disturbing symptoms would, for the sake of peace, be given a single room. Sometimes patients would be given single rooms only because no one would share with them or because they had been patients for longer than others and felt that they had a right to a single room. So a housing committee was formed to see what could be done. At first it consisted of delegates of patients and nursing staff; later, only patients were on the committee. Thus, apart from a small unit of seven beds under the direct control of the medical staff for physically sick patients, the patients themselves accepted the responsibility for deciding which beds new patients should occupy.

From that time onwards the situation improved. The patients dealt firmly with each other's attempts at gaining special attention through exploitation of symptoms, but at the same time were most helpful and understanding with really disturbed patients.

Representatives of the patient community attended, along with the cook and other kitchen and serving staff, the hospital catering meeting, held by the catering officer to discuss suggestions and complaints about menus, meal-times, and catering arrangements. Patient representatives also attended the medical director's weekly conference, which included other senior staff, to discuss problems that could not be satisfactorily solved at lower levels. Patients' advice was sought at departmental meetings on such topics as stoking, heating and hot water, economy in lighting, laundry bills, breakages, and so on. At one time there seemed to be a plethora of meetings, but as the hospital's new structure became established they became fewer in number.

The patients' meeting was subsequently held fortnightly, and its affairs were conducted by an elected committee of five. All matters arising were brought to the deputy matron daily by the executive members, this being the official link between patients and hospital authorities. Apart from this point of contact the patients' executive committee met the medical director, the principal administrative officer, and the matron every fortnight.

The topics discussed at the daily meetings of the patients' executive have ranged from mundane matters such as the shortage of teaspoons in the dining-room, electric irons out of order, and water not being hot enough, to sophisticated questions of management and the drawing up of a patients' constitution. The constitution contains one clause giving the executive members of the patients' meeting the responsibility for dealing with any behaviour that the community considers antisocial. Other clauses give guidance on matters of procedure. Whatever the problem, it is discussed in terms of what the patients can do about it themselves. It would often be easier for the staff to take the initiative, make a decision, or say what should be done, but staff are not omniscient, and may only perpetuate feelings of dependency or give little opportunity for patients to see what other ways there may be of solving difficulties.

The entertainments' committee flourished, providing entertainment when required, but it has become less necessary over the years. The advent of television has had no small effect in this sphere; furthermore, the patients have come increasingly to use entertainment facilities provided outside the hospital.

When the hospital was reorganized into four medical units, the housing committee as originally arranged was no longer required. Each medical unit decided for itself how it would manage its own affairs. Each unit now has its own housing committee and the patients continue to organize the bed allocation themselves.

The improved efficiency of patient organization in the separate medical units has had the effect of reducing interest in and attendance at the patients' total community meetings. This issue came to a head when attendance fell so low that the patients decided to discontinue the meetings for a time. However, after two months of inactivity, a number of patients formed themselves into a committee and called a meeting. The desire to maintain interest in total community affairs led the patients to meet fortnightly as before, and the executive committee to function again as the contact for the patients' total community with the hospital administration.[1]

This method of administration is useful in the Cassel Hospital and might be adapted to other situations; it does, however, produce its own difficulties. Not everyone likes responsibility; some people prefer to be dependent and to have other people talk for them and tell them what to do. Because of past experiences, many patients are suspicious of an authority that is not strong-armed, that does not *insist* that its particular ways of thinking or behaving must be right. And there are others who need to dominate situations at all costs or who try to exploit what they think to be weakness on the part of those in authority.

The skill of the leadership role in an organization such as this lies in knowing when to be active, when to make suggestions or take on a task oneself, when to point out the difficulty of the

[1] For later developments in the patients' community meetings, see Chapter 20 – Ed.

people concerned in taking responsibility and making decisions themselves. Sometimes ideas put forward by patients would mean extra work for staff. This is dealt with by saying: 'By all means have what you want, but how can you manage to arrange it from your own resources?' It is probably possible to show the patients what resources they have to deal with the problem, but at any rate the problem itself is back where it belongs – with the patients.

Inevitably, patients and staff are continually testing out a situation like this. Do the authorities, do the staff, do the patients, really mean what they say? How much will they stand? How far is it possible to go? By and large, the answers can be found if the following questions are asked: Who is really affected? Who bears the brunt of this decision? Can they in their turn deal with it adequately from their own resources?

A sample of the minutes of a patients' fortnightly general meeting now follows, with their permission. The names of the patients have been altered, to ensure anonymity.

MINUTES OF PATIENTS' MEETING, 2 FEBRUARY 1956[1]

A meeting was held, attended by sixteen patients, four members of the committee, and Sister Erikson. More patients arrived later.

Chairman	Mrs Brown
Vice-Chairman	Miss Jones
Secretary	—
Treasurer	Miss Smith
Fifth Member (Acting Sec.)	Miss Miller

The minutes of the previous meeting were read and confirmed. Matters listed below were discussed at the meeting.

Treasurer's report

Report read by chairman. Mrs Thoms commented that she thought there was a limit to the amount of the entertainments fund. Mr Johns said that anything in excess of £3 should be handed over to the sports and social fund. There were complaints that there was not enough money to run dances. It was agreed that not enough notice of dances was given, and improvements on the present

[1] Reprinted from the Cassel Hospital *Reports* for the five years 1 April 1953 to 31 March 1958, by kind permission of the management committee.

system of arranging dances were left to the new chairman and committee.

Mrs Thoms proposed, Mr Johns seconded, that anything in excess of £3 from the entertainments committee should be given to the sports and social fund:

16 in favour
1 against
6 abstained

Entertainments committee report

Mrs Bleak, the chairman, said that there was nothing to report. She read the treasurer's report, and suggested that notice of dances should be given one week ahead.

Mothers' report

Mrs Brown, the representative, mentioned a children's playroom. They were temporarily using an unused bedroom, but there was a children's teaching room which could be used, also temporarily, especially at week-ends. There were complaints that the children might spoil the room.

The meeting felt very strongly that a separate room exclusively for the use of children and their guardians was essential. Mrs Thoms proposed, Mr Johns seconded, that the hospital authorities should be again requested to provide a room for children, and the mothers would contribute some equipment to be kept there permanently:

22 in favour
1 abstained

Mr Johns remarked that Dr Main did not want a staff room used, but a patients' room.

(The meetings of 6 and 20 October discussed this same question with great feeling, the difficulty being solved because there was a spare room available which was offered as a playroom.)

Mrs Brown complained that adults wanted to watch other programmes while children's television was on. Miss Low said that children had priority during children's television time, and this was the feeling of the meeting in general. It was stressed that children, not adults, should have the right to choose which channel should be viewed. A proposal was made by Mr Gilbert, seconded by Mrs Thoms, that children should have priority during children's television time, but that they should not be in the television room unless in charge of a responsible adult. This was carried unanimously.

Mr Head said that a child had caused a disturbance during evening television. On further inquiry it was found that this incident involved a child running into the room and running out again. Mrs Brown said that the child had obviously escaped momentarily from his mother and that the remedy would be to turn the child out of the room. She could say, on behalf of the mothers, that this action would be welcomed.

Mr Gilbert said that children caused great disturbance in the dining-room. Mrs Brown said that the mothers would meet to discuss this, and would report to the next meeting.

Servery report

Mr Hand, the representative, said that a cloth was provided for cleaning the toaster, and requested that patients should use this instead of the tea cloth. Tea towels should be washed through on the 3–5 p.m. shift, and the unit responsible should boil them weekly. He suggested that patients who worked full time should do an occasional late-night tea duty. Miss Low suggested that each servery representative should make an official list of patients with regard to servery duties and check it with the sister. The question whether patients who did full-time work outside the hospital should also do servery duty was left over till the next meeting.

Mr Peak queried the patients' washing of tea towels. He wondered whether the staff tea towels were sent to the laundry, but no one knew. Miss Clear said that the patients' tea towels, at least, were sent to the laundry. Mr Peak proposed, Miss Mill seconded, that in the interest of hygiene, and in consideration of the fact that table cloths were not used (thus saving expense), we should protest against the decision that tea towels should not be sent to the laundry. This was carried unanimously.

Mr Hand continued that anyone who wanted to change servery duty should alter the list and inform reception. Mr Gilbert said that if someone was prepared to sign for the servery keys they should be given to him, even if his name was not on the list, and this should be mentioned to matron. When this was put to the vote there were fourteen in favour and seven abstentions. There were various objections and the chairman commented that a new arrangement was clearly required.

Patients who wanted early breakfast should put their names in the book before 4 p.m. The butter machine was to be replaced, and some of the patients requested a simpler kind of machine, but this was felt to be going too far ahead. A report book was to be placed in the servery for complaints about the previous shift. The meeting was unanimously in favour.

Servery inventory

Twenty-three teaspoons down, twenty trays missing, seventeen of the best blue cups short, thirty forks up (but still sixty down on the original number), fourteen mustard spoons found.

Mr Peak said that there should be 110 best blue cups, and proposed that enough new cups should be bought to bring the total up to a hundred in view of the original number. Mr East seconded, and the motion was carried unanimously.

Mr Johns complained of shortage of sugar in the last few days, and Mr Hare said that the tea ran out very quickly. Mr Hand said that he would put out more sugar, and would servery people please fill the urns right up with water.

Sports/social report

Mr Johns said that no meeting had been held. Mr Lord had bought a book of snooker rules for the hospital, and a vote of thanks was passed. He requested that the grand piano be repaired, and Mr East added that the other piano was also out of order again. These matters should be reported to the executive sisters of the relevant parts of the building.

Chairman's comments

Casting vote: the chairman brought up the question of whether the chairman should have a casting vote as well as an ordinary vote. Mr Johns proposed, Mr Peak seconded, that the chairman should have a casting vote but no other. This was carried unanimously except for two abstentions.

Water: The chairman reminded the meeting that patients should put in all wash-basin and bath plugs during frosty weather. Mr East said that the water could be turned off by a valve under the basin. Several patients said that this had caused flooding, and it was decided that the valve should not be touched; also that any leak should be reported straight away to a sister.

Wood: The chairman reported that some wood, left over from making swings, had been voted to be given free to Mr Bear who had previously gone to a lot of trouble over the swings.

Milk losses: in order to stop the considerable milk losses, the chairman suggested that one person from each unit should collect the appropriate amount of milk and take it to the unit's rooms, which would isolate any losses. Some patients thought that this was unnecessary, and it was left to be decided at unit level. Mrs Stair reported that her unit had already started to use this method and found it very satisfactory.

(The meeting still being in progress at 9.16 p.m., the late tea in the servery was retarded by fifteen minutes.)

Page-numbering: The chairman mentioned that Sister Thomas had asked for volunteers to help with the page-numbering of a lecture report. Work could be collected from Miss Finkin's office at any time of the day, and the necessary equipment and information would be given for this simple and straightforward job.

Facilities: The chairman read out a letter signed by Mrs Thoms, in which she said: 'In view of the fact that our unit is large and the facilities are barely adequate for our needs, coupled with the fact that young babies are housed in the unit and therefore disturbance is to be avoided, it has been decided by the members of the unit that *all* the facilities within the unit, including the quiet room, will in future be for the use of unit patients only. Following the above decision, we hereby return the sum of £1 recently allocated to us by the sports and social fund for the purchase of various items of kitchen equipment for use in the unit kitchen.'

Mr Johns stated that the previous inhabitants of that unit had been more generous with their facilities than the present ones. The chairman observed that the quiet room in the unit had been the only one in the hospital, and quiet study should surely not cause disturbance to the young babies as had been feared. It was stated that the typewriter was noisy, but the suggestion that it could be used in the unit office, leaving the quiet room for study, was not taken up. On the chairman inquiring to whom the typewriter belonged, Mr Gilbert replied, 'To the sisters.'

Mr Head suggested that the work room typewriter should be locked in a cupboard, but it was felt that it would be sufficient if it were merely put away in one, when not in use, out of the children's way. Mr Gilbert interposed here that the cupboards be moved to another wall to make more room for billiards, but it was decided to defer this to another meeting.

Crockery

Mrs Thoms reiterated that crockery should not be left in the common room, which her unit had to keep clean and tidy. In future the unit would undertake to remove none of it and would let it pile up there.

Telephones

The GPO had complained that the patients' telephone had remained unanswered one afternoon, causing delay over the delivery of a telegram. Would patients be more ready to answer the phone, especially if it was very persistent, since it could well be a matter of urgency. One telephone was out of order, which could have caused the delay, but this would be remedied. It was further requested that the condition of the two pianos be looked into.

Watch committee

The chairman said that the patients' executive committee was normally required to act as a watch committee to check any immoral behaviour on the part of patients. Miss Lark suggested having a separate committee, but it was decided to hold an extraordinary meeting on the following Monday to discuss this subject exclusively.

Losses

As it was getting late, the question of recent losses was deferred until the next patients' meeting.

Catering representatives

Mr Sands volunteered to be catering representative on the retirement of Mrs Tetley.

Complaint

Mrs Pain suggested that patients who did not contribute to the television fund should not be allowed to vote when a choice of programmes was made.

The chairman proposed, Miss Miller seconded, that the names of the people who paid should be put on a board in the television room, and that the patients not on this list could not vote in the choice of programmes:

5 in favour
3 against
3 abstained

The proposal was carried.

It was decided to postpone the elections until the next meeting, since nearly all the patients had gone out to get tea, and it was very cold in the committee room.

The chairman declared the meeting closed.

It is not, of course, possible to make people go to meetings unless you are prepared to take police action and impose penalties for non-attendance. If you did this, the amount of hostility aroused would probably nullify the usefulness of the meetings. However, when there is a need, when something urgently requires a settlement, people will usually get together for that purpose. Sometimes meetings are avoided as a way of shelving a difficult matter, and this may go on for some time. But as long as the opportunity exists for such meetings to take place, they tend to be fruitfully used when the occasion demands.

9 · *Patient–Staff Activities in Medical Units*

BY E. JEANETTE GAZDAR

Each of the four medical units comprises a group of patients, a porter, a cleaner, a senior sister, trainee nurses, and two or three doctors, all under the supervision of a full- or part-time consultant and responsible for a certain area of the hospital. Each unit formulates its own policy for administration, for the selection, admission, and treatment of patients, and for the meetings and discussions it will hold. There is an overall expectation that patients will take part in the daily work of the unit.

Patients are responsible for making their beds, for the general care and cleanliness of their rooms, and for assisting the porter and cleaner in the daily cleaning of the various public rooms and corridors in their unit areas, between the hours of 9 a.m. and 12 noon. Each unit patient group holds a weekly works meeting conducted by a patient chairman, or 'works manager', and attended by all the patients (except those working outside the hospital) and by the nursing staff and cleaner. Work is allocated to new patients by the works manager, or reallocated to other patients, just as the patient housing representative allocates beds and rooms to new patients, with help or advice from the staff when the need arises. There is an opportunity for problems to be discussed and complaints to be ventilated.

The matron supplies all non-fixed equipment and materials for internal decoration. She allocates an annual sum of money to each unit so that it can arrange its own interior decoration, and obtain replacements of linen, furniture, and other equipment as required, within this budget. Opportunities are given for patients to express their ideas about all these things and to take part in choosing patterns, colours, materials, and so on. Patients then appreciate the need to consider the costs of the services they are using.

PROBLEMS OF CO-OPERATION

Certain services may be provided by a unit for the total community: one provides the dining-room and servery service, completely undertaken by patients, and another a combined staff and patient kitchen service.

The servery and dining-room service has undergone four changes since the days when it was provided solely by staff. As an experiment we asked patients to help at peak hours during times of staff sickness and holidays, and this seemed quite successful. Then, as staff members left they were not replaced, but patients went to help during each shift of duty. This latter arrangement was not liked by the staff, who felt their jobs to be in jeopardy; also, they felt strongly that they could not work with patients who failed to appear regularly for work, selected the jobs they wanted to do, were untidy and dirty by staff standards, disappeared when they got bored, and left the brunt of the work to a reduced staff. They felt frustrated that they were no longer able to maintain their former high standard of cleanliness and efficiency. Patients complained of the staff attitude and were equally unhappy in the situation. Nursing staff members tried hard to link the two sections, but without success.

Eventually, the patients of one unit were given complete responsibility for providing servery service for all patients, and the staff were transferred to a smaller servery to cater for all staff. The staff group settled down happily in its new surroundings, but the patients' problems increased with their greater responsibilities. They had to arrange shift rotas, cope with members who failed to return dirty dishes from their rooms, and with those who filched food (some patients have particular difficulties in this respect). After many vicissitudes some measure of satisfaction was achieved. The next thing was that a member of the medical staff of the unit providing the servery service left the hospital for another post. This meant that there were fewer patients in the unit and they were no longer able to manage the work. Appeals for help sent to other units met initially with little response. Finally, the senior sister of the unit arranged a meeting at which it was agreed by the patients that each medical unit would participate in the service by undertaking responsibility for it on certain days of the week.

The kitchen service presented fewer difficulties, no doubt because the cooks did not feel that they would be ousted by patients; the kitchen maids, though not too easy about it at first, gradually accepted having patients working with them. The head cook has become increasingly more appreciative of patient help, on which she is very dependent during staff holidays, and those most interested now assist her with cake- and pastry-making. The patients, particularly the women, are usually rather hesitant to work in the kitchen, whereas the men regard it as a novelty and are by and large more popular with the staff. Work for men in the hospital is a real problem, since there are relatively few tasks that a man would normally undertake. Getting work outside the hospital is not always easy, though local firms and officers of the labour exchange are most helpful.

In the medical units, problems arising between staff and patients, or between patients, are dealt with by the parties concerned meeting together to thrash them out. Where possible a policy is decided on and action indicated. Sometimes a recommendation has to be taken to another unit or department of the hospital and, again, the people affected will meet together to see what can be done. With a clear administrative structure it is fairly easy to see who should get together with whom about a particular problem. For instance, the hospital provides laundry facilities for patients, a room equipped with a washing machine, deep sinks, drying and airing cupboards, wringer, boiler, and irons. The care and cleanliness of this room is the responsibility of one of the medical units. The hot-water supply, on the other hand, is the concern of the principal administrative officer of the hospital. Soon after the installation of the washing machine the patients complained that it was useless because there was no hot water. These complaints came up at the patients' meetings in the units and were referred back to the unit responsible for providing the service. The senior sister of that unit together with patient representatives then discussed the matter with the administrative officer. One of the patients concerned happened to know quite a lot about hot-water systems and his suggestions were useful.

A lot of talk goes on in this kind of nursing, but it is out in the open. Some kind of decision is usually reached and action initiated by mutual agreement; even if it is only decided to do nothing for the time being, everyone knows how and why that decision was reached.

10 · *The Nursing Approach to a Family*

BY IRENE GLEESON

To find out what a patient's illness means to the family and how far the family can be helped to keep together were matters of special emphasis when it was first proposed to admit a young mother and her baby to the Cassel Hospital.

We were asked by a welfare clinic to admit the mother, who was in great difficulty with her six-week-old baby; she had severe fears of harming him, and of not feeding him properly and not giving him enough. She was distraught when he cried and felt a complete failure as a mother. She suffered from panic states and could not bear to be left alone in her flat with the child. This affected her husband, who could go to work only if assured that the health visitor or some kindly neighbour would stay with his wife.

As the nurse responsible for the admission of new patients to this particular medical unit, I went to see this family and, with my consultant's authority, offered admission to the mother and the baby. It seemed to me that the mother regarded this as an ideal solution but that the husband, though willing to fall in with any plans for his wife's improvement, was rather depressed about the whole idea. He felt that his wife and son were being taken from him (albeit by kindly people) and that he himself had no part to play in her recovery. I got the impression that relationships in the home were fairly strained and that the separation of these two people might eventually be harmful to the marriage.

As a result of this home visit, the patient's doctor decided to offer the husband accommodation in the hospital – at first for week-ends only. The two were given a double room, allocated to them by the patients' housing committee (not without curiosity and foreboding, for this was a new departure), and the husband came for three nights weekly as a guest. He paid for his meals as do other patients' guests. This arrangement was later extended to include holiday periods, and the husband took part in the hospital activities, including the work. This proved to be quite a good arrangement because the mother was much less anxious with the child when her husband was with her. The husband was able to reassure himself almost daily that things were not so bad. The situation brought to light many of the couple's difficulties with each other which had not been acknowledged by either of them, and this was helpful in the patient's treatment. Eventually they moved out to their new house, as a family.

ACCOMMODATING THE FAMILY IN HOSPITAL

When admitting a mother and her child now, we try to offer accommodation to the husband. This is not always accepted by the husband, but it usually is. If there are older children of school age who cannot be accommodated in the hospital, the mother is encouraged to bring them into the hospital as often as possible or to see them at home. Several times we have been able to house a whole disturbed family, father, mother, and children, for a holiday period, when some patients go away and we have vacant beds. This housing of the family helps greatly in maintaining the link with the home.

The patients in this particular medical unit become uneasy from time to time about the admission of families and on several occasions have voiced their fear of being swamped by too many of them. They seek reassurance that they will not be sent away in favour of more families. However, the housing committee, elected by the patients themselves, now regards family status as the criterion for the more desirable accommodation. Previously, length of stay in the hospital had been the qualifying condition.

Pre-admission visits to the patients' homes have helped in determining the advisability of separating the patient from the family. (So far we have concentrated on visiting mothers of young children before admission.) There is not only the family requesting help to be considered, but quite often the in-laws as well, especially when there is a new baby in the family.

In certain circumstances, therefore, the aim is to admit the family to hospital, not just one member. Of course, it is not possible to provide sleeping accommodation for the whole family but it is possible to provide an environment where the family can meet daily in the fairly ordinary atmosphere of a community which presents many of the responsibilities and privileges to be found in life outside hospital.

By expecting from the beginning that the family will continue to own and support its sick member, with the temporary help of the hospital staff and their technical skill, one can increase the possibility of maintaining family unity and ease the difficulty to the patient and the family of the return home.

11 · *When a Patient Leaves Hospital*

BY GILLIAN W. ELLES

It is useful to look at the occasion when a patient leaves hospital from the point of view of the patient and from the point of view of the group he is leaving, and to examine the relationship between these two. Many patients are able during their stay in hospital to assume a greater degree of freedom and responsibility than they were accustomed to in their own homes or at work before admission. Each one about to be discharged has to consider what he is leaving behind and what sort of home or job he is going to, and the two are linked by his feelings, his hopes and fears.

The unit in which I worked had fifteen patients, between twenty and forty years of age; married and single, men and women. Some had been in hospital before, others had not. The unit had two nurses, myself and a colleague. Recently this group of seventeen people had taken over responsibility for a new area in the hospital. Much of the work together had been centred on this task. It was at this point that six of the most active members of the group were ready for discharge, having been in hospital for about four months.

Each of the six had his own individual problems in leaving the hospital and going back to the situation in which he had originally become ill. With the nurse these patients had to face the realization that they were not completely symptom free, and the anxiety of wondering whether they would be able to carry on as they wanted to outside the hospital. At the same time, there were distinct difficulties of a practical nature relating to home or to work for which they had to find a solution. The problems of three of these six patients will illustrate the nature of the nursing tasks.

One of the patients was a young man of twenty-six who had never lived away from home. The nurse had met his mother and understood to some extent not only the patient's problem of leaving home, but also the mother's problem of making it possible for him to go. This made it easier for her to help this man to decide to find rooms for himself away from home, and to reassure his mother.

The second patient, a young woman wishing on the one hand for a professional career and on the other for a life in the country, was able to discuss with her nurse which of the two she might follow. The decision ultimately was hers, but with the nurse she was able to explore what she could hope to get out of each, both in terms of immediate satisfaction and in terms of long-range goals. The nurse to begin with did not know what the expectations were in either case; therefore she and the patient collaborated to find out more about the technical details, which helped the patient to make her decision.

The third patient was a married man who had been unable to work for several years and whose wife, as a result of his illness, had had to become the breadwinner. She now had a highly successful career, and was providing all they could want materially. However, the situation highlighted the sense of failure felt by the patient. Both he and his wife were able to discuss separately with the nurse the problems arising out of this, as well as the man's own problem of having been discharged from other hospitals before, only to become sick again. The fact that the nurse could allow the patient to discuss with her his uncertainty about keeping well this time seemed to be quite important to him.

With a number of people leaving at one time, some of whom were the unit's most able members, it was obvious that the work of the unit was going to be affected. These were the people who had done the pioneer work when the unit took over the new area. The unit, therefore, had to face what was going to happen once they had gone. At various works meetings attended by the patients under their own chairman, with the two nurses present, those who were leaving agreed to train others to take their place as key members. In return, patients who were staying on were able to offer help to those who were leaving. People going for interviews for jobs would often be accompanied by another patient who was not leaving.

One patient thought that she was going to have to refurnish her flat, and members in the group who could sew offered to help her with the curtains. It seemed that the unit at this point had undertaken a dual task: to make sure that the work should go on as smoothly as possible, and to help people to leave in a way that gave them confidence to carry on successfully. It was at this point that the nursing in the unit seemed to alter, and the roles of staff and patients merged in order that the group could work as a whole towards this twofold purpose.

Finally, a third problem arose. People who were leaving became very sensitive about the fact that a number of patients in the hospital were having a more lengthy treatment than they had had. Did this mean that the leavers were better or worse, more or less stable, or more liked or disliked than others in the hospital? The group sought to deal with this problem by having a long discussion among themselves about it. They examined hopes and fears about leaving while still having some symptoms. They considered their feelings of dependency on the hospital, their anxiety about being asked to leave. At the same time the patients remaining were able to look at some of the difficulties arising out of not going: whether they felt themselves envious of those able to go, or guilty that they were able to stay. It was as a result of this discussion that the group remained an active one to the end, and both those staying and those leaving were able to gain from the group's examination of the problems of having to adapt to change.

This experience in which a third of the patient group left at the same time produced three types of nursing problem. First, there were the problems relating to individual patients. Sometimes the nursing staff did not know the sort of information that might be useful to particular patients. Often all they did was to collaborate with the individual and sometimes with other patients to find a way of finding out. Second, time was limited, yet they found demands on it increasing. As a result the nursing became shared throughout the group, as did the work tasks. Third, as a group we all had to share the anxiety of these patients who were about to be discharged from hospital, and try to help them to maintain their relationships with people in the hospital, as well as to assist them to renew relationships outside.

Those who remained in the hospital also had to cope with absorbing new patients into a group that had just seen one-third of its members leave. The new patients needed to feel that they belonged to a group and could help in the work of the unit, if they were to be able to make use of what the hospital offered.

12 · *Some Costs of Neurotic Breakdown*

BY GILLIAN W. ELLES

The benefits to a nation of an efficient health service are obvious enough for medical treatment to be reckoned a wise national investment. Nevertheless, the high financial cost of the treatment services alarms many people, raising the question whether the most costly illnesses justify the money spent on them. A relatively quick, cheap, life-saving surgical operation such as an appendicectomy offers considerable financial benefits to the individual, his family, and the labour force of the nation. The corresponding value of long, expensive treatments for chronic or recurring illnesses can be in some doubt. There are many arguments but few facts to help us in this matter, for very little is known of the costs of *not* treating such conditions.

This paper reports an exploratory investigation into some costs of severe neurotic breakdown, and some of the costs of treatment. The direct financial outlay on the treatment of neurotic illness is not too difficult to estimate, but attempts to assess treatment as an investment are misleading if based only on the actual and obvious expenditure of money. The *social* costs of neurosis, in terms of family disruption, lowering of work status, limitations of mobility, are considerable in some cases and not easy to assess in financial terms; the *psychological* costs, in terms of uncertain mental economy, lack of internal emotional balance, personal restrictions, are equally difficult to evaluate and may be the most significant of all for the patient.

RESEARCH PLAN

Thirty-nine cases of severe neurotic breakdown were studied in depth. They were divided into two series, an initial pilot study of fourteen and a representative sample of twenty-five, drawn from the hospital population. The collected information was assessed in terms of various gains and losses, financial, social, and psychological. Particular attention was paid to those nuances of individual and family behaviour in order to estimate more accurately the gains and losses of illness and treatment.

The first idea was to try to reduce these accounts to a common financial denominator in order to compare one case with another. The research showed, however, that it could not express exactly what is the value of a life lived fully. It also highlighted the fact that human transactions of profit and loss occur at many levels. The 'currencies' for services of looking after the sick can be quoted in terms of *money*, *obligation*, and *affection*. These 'currencies' are not exactly convertible into one another, but the 'cost' quoted in one is directly linked to the costs of the other two.

The case-material was that of severe neurosis, sometimes with psychotic pathology, regarded by the treating doctors as requiring hospital treatment and intensive psychotherapy, with a poor prognosis for full recovery. The very admission to hospital showed that the family, general practitioner, outpatient psychiatry, friends, workmates, employers, and the patients themselves had not been able to cope. Some patients had a long history of various treatments elsewhere. All had one common feature, with its own prognostic and financial import – a readiness to abandon home, friends, and work in order to enter hospital.

PILOT STUDY

Fourteen patients discharged during the year 1955–6, who lived within easy reach of the hospital, were selected in March 1957 for the pilot study. At least twelve months had elapsed since their discharge, time enough to show significant trends towards rehabilitation and recent enough for the ex-patients to be well remembered by the clinical team. Their experiences represented various aspects of the problems of costing we wanted to explore and, with their help, methods were established of collecting data for analysis. They were approached not as clinical cases who might need further help but as respondents who could give useful information. Preliminary approach was by letter, in the hope of an invitation to visit them at home. Two early replies showed uneasiness at the prospect of a visit, whereafter each approach letter was accompanied by a questionnaire which the ex-patient was invited to return completed if a home visit was unwelcome. The questionnaire seemed to reassure the ex-patients about our intentions and there were few subsequent objections to home visits. Most patients seemed eager to contribute and glad to be remembered by the hospital.

When agreement to a home visit was obtained, one or more visits were made. Detailed information was sought from the patient and his family about his present state of health, the manifest financial costs of the breakdown, and the non-financial costs of it on his family. An outline of the pattern of social adaptation following discharge was based on this information and on observations made by the worker.

Similar information was also sought, by letter and interview, from the hospital doctor, general practitioner, and any doctor still treating the patient. Information given by the general practitioner posed problems of financial costing. *The per capita charge of the national health service in no way corresponds to the extra work and strain these patients often caused their doctors.* The patients' employers were not approached and relevant information was derived from family sources.

The approach to patients could not be standardized. All correspondence and interviewing had to be timed and tailored to fit each case. The search for corroboratory detail also required contacts with other people and other hospitals.

The 'costing' scheme covered general family history, family activity, structure of the home, superficial health survey of the family. The changes in each of these associated with the patient's breakdown were worked out against a background of family history and aspirations. Where possible, the changes were described from the point of view of the patient, other significant relatives, and the general practitioner. Where financial costing was used, all costs and gains were adjusted to those obtaining for the year 1955–6.

THE MAIN STUDY

Following the pilot study of patients living near to the hospital, it was decided to pursue these accounting attempts with a representative sample of the hospital intake for the same year. Every fourth patient on an alphabetical list of discharges was selected, giving twenty-five names. On examination, this small group was found to be representative of the usual age range, sex distribution, marital status, and diagnoses of patients of the previous five years: it consisted of eight men and seventeen women; five of the men were married, three with children, two without, and three were single; five of the women were married, three with children, two without, two were widowed, and ten were single.

More difficulty was encountered in the initial contact. Two patients were not seen personally, one was too ill and the other did not speak English. The psychiatrists treating them were interviewed instead. Another patient could not be traced, but information from her general practitioner and those with whom she lived was readily available. Three women had just had babies and were protected by a ring of supportive relatives and general practitioners. Much information was volunteered through correspondence, however. Two men refused a home visit, though one, met by chance on a train, was only too ready to discuss his progress.

For the sample patients, the research evaluation of treatment was compared with the hospital doctor's evaluation at the point of discharge two years previously, and with a postal survey conducted by the hospital a year later (*Table 1*).

TABLE 1 RESULTS OF TREATMENT

Time of rating	*MI*	*I*	*NC*	*W*	*MW*	*C*	*U*	*Total*
On discharge	3	11	9	1	–	–	1	25
1 year later (postal survey)	7	4	2	3	–	–	9	25
Research follow-up	10	10	2	2	–	1	–	25

MI = much improved; I = improved; NC = no change; W = worse; MW = much worse; C = circular; U = unrated.

DEFINITIONS AND LIMITATIONS

'Breakdown'

It must be emphasized that all the cases examined were not merely of 'neurotic illness' but of manifest, hospitalized neurotic *breakdown*, with collapse of working ability, finances, and, sometimes, social and family relationships. Even these postulates do not fully define all the cases. Some had prior history of long inactivity at home, clearly neurotic but disguised by family adaptations and special arrangements. While this prior period was not one of breakdown, not including it in the costing would have been misleading. The study became concerned with the balance between financial and social costs of manifest neurotic breakdown involving hospitalization and of neurotic patterns before breakdown involving maladapted behaviour which resulted in isolation, ostracism, idleness, and financial dependency.

Failure to find a single yardstick for estimating costs

Costs were arranged in three periods of time – before, during, and after hospitalization – and were divided between the individual, the family, the employer, and the state. This tabulation led to the conclusion that *financial cost varies less with the character and intensity of the illness than with the capacity of the home to absorb the illness without seeking help from the social services.*

'Costs' thus emerges as a relative and inexact term, sometimes expressed in clear, financial transactions and sometimes in terms of family effort or personal distress. A married woman with children tended to assess her problems in essentially emotional terms whereas an unmarried woman would draw attention also to financial losses in salary and pension rights. The men, both married and single, referred more directly to financial losses than did the women, but for them money often had more than cash value and seemed to reflect emotional problems of status as well. One man hesitated to reveal his low salary because he felt it to be an index of failure, though his family and doctor thought he had made a good recovery. Problems of prestige, status at work, and actual salary were important to the men, whereas the satisfactory nature of the home, which might include the occupational status of the husband or fiancé, was more important to the women.

Some families assessed the severity of the illness and the effect of treatment in terms of work, meaning money, and those who classed themselves as 'working class' used this yardstick almost to the exclusion of any other. 'He must be all right, he's working', would be the attitude. Other costs, even of great family unhappiness and inefficiency, were largely discounted. If the patient wage-earner himself emphasized other costs, such as personal strain or difficulties in social relations, this would be out of step with the family assessment. Financial, family, individual, and medical yardsticks were not only different but sometimes contradictory.

Limitation of financial yardstick

Following treatment, some married men earned less than before their illness but made important non-financial gains of greater value to their lives. One patient who led an unhappy life at home, who could not get on with his in-laws, and whose wife worked hard while he was inefficient in a skilled job, altered his pattern following treatment. He got a less well-paid job for which he was better fitted, his marriage improved, his wife stopped working when she became pregnant, and he got on better with his in-laws, who then gave him a job in the family business. These linked events cost £500 in one year but brought greater happiness and security for the patient and his family. The importance to them of reconnecting with the wider family structure was that they were now fulfilling more mature aspirations of marriage and family relationships. There was no conflict, at individual or family level, about accepting a smaller salary. In those families where money is the yardstick, however, such a solution would have caused greater anxiety for the family.

Money can be used as a substitute, albeit incomplete, for good relationships. Financial success as an alternative to 'affective currency' (ability to maintain constancy in relationships) was seen in the case of a married woman who went back to her career and relinquished her family responsibilities. She is now earning well but her relationships are impoverished and unsatisfactory to her. Cut off from people who cared for her, she risks another breakdown, and it is likely in the future that the health service may have to pay out much on her account. Such expenditure could be regarded in a general sense as the *financial equivalent of recreative and therapeutic relationships of family and community* which cannot be enjoyed by this patient.

Unsuccessful search for a universal basis for computation

Overall costing in financial terms was made impossible, in practice, by the different yardsticks used by the patients and others interviewed. The question, 'Was the cost of treatment worth it?', is equally difficult to answer precisely because of the apparent impossibility of converting one 'currency' into another. In estimating improvement, however, it became apparent that *all 'currencies' must somehow be given their full weight.*

Some non-financial yardsticks for assessing the effects of treatment

For married people an important yardstick concerned the success or failure of maintaining a triad of relationships – with the family of procreation, the family of origin, and at work. Earning money was certainly one way of enriching and maintaining these, but to earn affection and privilege was equally important. For the unmarried, success or failure at home and at work were similarly important, but the third area of relationships making the stabilizing triad was that of their peer group. Such single items as 'medical recovery' were misleading. For no patient did one single yardstick, financial or other, really express the true profit and loss. Again, 'work performance and earnings' would alone provide an insufficient indication of the effects of treatment or the patient's capacity to maintain improvement. Some families were prepared to use this one yardstick, however.

The importance of the family in deciding the major 'currency'

The patient's psychopathology may play the major part in deciding the success or failure of his relationships but it does not necessarily decide who bears the cost of the failure, or whether this is experienced in terms of money, social standing, or emotional burden. In the sample, *the family structure much governed the final choice of 'currency' and who paid it.*

This supportive family structure depended upon key members of the family incorporating within themselves a pattern of family functioning which derived in part from an *actual* experience of family strength and in part from a good-enough relationship with people who had cared for them in such a family, usually their own parents. There were three main patterns that could be incorporated. First, there was the pattern of the family with a longstanding experience of prospering and of being able to care for both the very young and the infirm. Second, there was the family that did not have a longstanding experience of a cultural pattern. Family members were very much in touch with each other's needs and feelings. Such a pattern gave less security during moments of crisis than the first one, having little sense of historical process. Finally, there were families operating by a 'family ordained myth' which required family members to enact certain roles and to hold certain views of life in order to remain part of the family. In these, individual perceptions became subservient to the family way of seeing life, and the security such families offered was a costly one, leading to family members' withdrawing from other groups. These three types of 'inner' family structure deeply affected the deployment of the available resources.

The supporting capacity of the family was seen in some cases to be a national economic resource of immense value, limiting direct financial outlay on welfare, hospital, and health services, helping the patient to retain social relationships, and, through tolerance of deviant behaviour, limiting the development of those secondary features of severe neurotic illness which spring from individual isolation, 'anomie', and from uncaring or punitive reactions by an uninvolved community. The study suggests that the capacity of the family to adjust to the needs of its neurotic member is at best advantage when it operates as a unit of three generations. Family roles can be split or reallocated with considerable flexibility, lessening the emotional and social impoverishment that might ensue in the nuclear family or in isolated individuals. Where the supporting capacity of the family was poor, the cost more quickly assumed financial forms to be borne by others.

Examples of remedial family activity in operation were provided by cases in which the patients were married men with children. They tended, less than the childless men, to rely on their wives' earning capacity and they returned to work more quickly. At first, it seemed that this might be only a response to fatherhood but later it was seen that wider family influences were at work. Because they had children, these patients got more help from parents and parents-in-law than did the childless. Neighbourhood ties acted more in their favour. The children, by altering the family structure and its position in the community, affected the length of the illness and the types of cost, both the manner in which they appeared and the way in which they were apportioned.

Up to the point of breakdown, a family could bear many costs in hidden form. It could assume domestic responsibilities, in the interests of lessening the tension but at the cost of limiting another's personal freedom. In such unobtrusive ways, a family can pay heavily for its patient's illness. It seems that the patient is declared 'broken down' when the family feels the price too great to be borne and repudiates its task. It was at this point that *responsibility for bearing the illness was transferred to the hospital or social services*, and the costs, hitherto hidden in and borne by the family, could now be quoted in terms of financial outlay. In short, the cost of treatment appeared to be the monetary equivalent of family relationships which had failed, and hospitalization reflected the condition of the family as much as that of the patient. Where family breakdown was quickly reached, the cost more readily assumed financial forms.

WAS TREATMENT WORTH IT?

The survey suggests that if the national health service had not undertaken the treatment of these cases of severe neurotic breakdown, and had thus saved overt financial cost, somebody else, probably the family, would have faced the bill in silent, more or less stressful, rearrangements, even by illness. The cost of this risk to a family cannot be excluded from any true reckoning of the results or value of medical treatment. Similarly, the gains and losses to an employer and to the labour force of the nation are essential data if the results of treatment are to be truly assessed.

Lacking a satisfactory universal basis for computing the cost of illness, the study could only suggest that in the total cost of breakdown the cost of the restrictions imposed on others is not necessarily less than the financial cost of the hospital services. The big, closely knit family is, however, better able to apportion these costs. It is clear that if a period of treatment in hospital can benefit a family system, either partially or wholly, temporarily or permanently, then it is worth much. It seems likely that if, in assessments of the results of treatment, less emphasis were to be laid on symptomatic recovery (the medical yardstick) and more on those yardsticks by which *the individual and his family* will measure improvement, a re-evaluation of the effects of psychiatric treatment would occur. It was noteworthy in this study how the hospital doctors, using perhaps perfectionist criteria, tended to be less satisfied with the results of their treatment than were the patients or their families. They were, legitimately, measuring different things, but, in terms of benefit to the patient and family, the latter's view needs to be better known and taken into account by hospital staff.

ESTIMATING COSTS

The following factors were found to give the most accurate estimation of the total cost of neurotic breakdown:

1. length of invalidism
2. type of isolation of individual and family
3. type of work loss
4. pattern of transfer of living expenses
5. pattern of transfer of role tasks, privileges, and responsibilities.

In each of the above there is a personal and a social element because the individual's loss of social capacity is one determinant, and society's capacity to respond is another. In all the cases reviewed there was a combination of different types of costs, which could be classified as:

6. actual financial costs
7. restricted relationships
8. personal distress
9. social dislocation.

The smallest units of cost, resulting in either loss or gain, were of 'membership units', i.e. family and family member, firm and employee, health service and patient.

Family/family member costs were seen to include loss of earnings plus extra home costs associated with the breakdown, and also such items as loss of fundamental capacity to work, with its attendant feeling of deep failure, and all the social impoverishment and isolation. These effects, in many cases, involved the whole family, and the gravity of the situation depended not only on the presence of the sick person in the family, but also on the stability of the family and the vigour of the community.

In the main study, which contained thirteen single and twelve married patients (including two widowed), ten single patients appeared to have emotionally disturbed parents, and eleven married patients appeared to have unstable partners. The data suggest that the sickest person may not be the 'patient', that the 'patient' may be the one most able to tolerate change, and that between neurotic couples there exists a benign complementarity, which only in stress situations shows either as individual neurotic breakdown or as total family disturbance.

Firm/employee costs were difficult to assess with accuracy, because in only very few cases was it possible to hear the opinions of the employer or work associates. Loss of opportunity for promotion did not accompany sickness absence from semi-skilled work, though the sickness benefits in such cases were limited to standard payments of usually a third to a half of one year's salary. Skilled workers often had longer periods of sick pay, especially if linked with long service, but the standard of mental health required on return was more exacting, and therefore an intervening period of rehabilitation more costly.

Health service/patient costs varied, showing at one end of the scale patterns of relatively 'cheap' treatment associated with little or no opportunity for paid work or marriage (e.g. the long-stay chronic wards) and, at the other, 'expensive' treatment aiming at rehabilitation to gainful work and home life. Where the cost per bed was high but the treatment enabled the patient to reach these goals, the total cost in the long run may be *less* than the aggregate cost of the 'cheap' hospital costs without realistic home and work achievements. State organizations were used earlier for isolated patients who needed domestic care as well as treatment. Therefore all treatment costs had to be carefully scrutinized for inclusive 'cost of living', which often had to be paid as part of the cost of effective therapy, but which could not accurately be described as part of the cost of breakdown, only as part of the cost of being alive. This cost of living was seen as something that was transferred in times of illness, and *the network of the transfers appeared more important in assessing the gravity of the illness and the problem of rehabilitation than did the financial costs involved.*

There follow two examples, one of a single woman and one of

a married woman, which show how the above factors were applied in the survey.

Miss A., aged 31

Original diagnosis:	severe obsessional neurosis
Age at breakdown:	20
1. Length of invalidism:	12 years; 39 per cent of life
2. Type of isolation:	completely dependent on family; withdrawal into home; parents elderly and isolated, daughter's illness isolates them further; no friends; no work; two short spells in hospital
3. Type of work loss:	bank clerk before breakdown, £250 per annum
(*a*) work pattern before illness:	2 years' work; difficult social relationships affect competence
(*b*) work pattern after breakdown:	unemployment; withdrawal into home without assuming any responsibility in home
(*c*) calculated work loss:	over 10 years, £3,850; job had top salary of £570, with pension of £380 after 20 years
(*d*) present work:	unskilled work as lift attendant
(*e*) relation to family's work pattern:	present job below expectations but seen as improvement; unlikely to be in family's social class (father was bank manager)
4. Transfer of living expenses:	father on pension, provides comfortable home; mother and 'daily' provide care; way of life not changed
5. Transfer of role tasks, privileges, responsibilities	
During breakdown:	
(*a*) wage-earner	to father, now on pension
(*b*) daughter role in home	suspended except when mother went to hospital, twice

(*c*) peer group member role	makes one friend in hospital, keeps on discharge
(*d*) community member role	only through parents and their contacts

During recovery:

(*a*) wage-earner	reinvested in self
(*b*) daughter role in home	begins to reinvest
(*c*) peer group member role	not developed
(*d*) community member role	not developed

6. Actual financial costs:

(*a*) through invalidism	£3,396[1]	£7,246
(*b*) through loss of work	£3,850	

7–9. Restricted relationships, personal distress, social dislocation:	no friends; no security; no community status except through parents; loss of marriage opportunity; loss of work skills

Mrs B., aged 39

Original diagnosis:	phobic anxieties and depression
Age at breakdown:	33
Health of family:	husband, narcolepsy; son 1, insomnia and anxiety away from home; son 2, nocturnal enuresis
1. Length of invalidism:	6 years (1 of treatment); 15 per cent of life
Continuation of invalidism after treatment:	2 years
2. Type of isolation:	cannot leave house, other members not isolated; depends on husband's and

[1] The costs of invalidism were assessed as follows:

(i) Known family expenses	– food, housing, clothes, pocket money	£1,716
	– private psycho-analysis	£1,050
(ii) State expenses	– hospital costs	£ 630

	children's co-operation; cannot drive car; on bad terms with parents and in-laws; no social life except through children's friends
3. Type of work loss:	stopped work when first pregnant; hates staying at home; cannot shop by herself; domestic chores seen as Herculean tasks
4. Transfer of living expenses:	(*a*) to husband at first pregnancy (*b*) to hospital at breakdown (*c*) to husband on discharge
5. Transfer of role tasks, privileges, responsibilities	
Before treatment:	
(*a*) mothering	to husband
(*b*) housekeeper	self (unwilling)
(*c*) professional worker in middle-class setting	suspended, envious of husband's ability

Factors 6–9 (actual financial costs, restricted relationships, personal distress, and social dislocation) can only be assessed together because they are highly interrelated:

Mrs B. found hospital admission a great relief. It meant a return to a middle-class, liberal *milieu* which, through giving up her career and marrying a man unable to provide the desired status, she had lost. Her family developed an extended structure while she was in hospital, mother and mother-in-law ran the home and the children's isolation was reduced. On her discharge, however, she again isolated the family through her own social difficulties which treatment had not altered.

Actual financial costs of hospital treatment were about £1,000. Total expenditure will only partly be paid by the 'presenting patient'. The children are probably deeply affected by the uneasy parental relationship and by the clumsy way in which the parents handle their social relationships. This case, then, is very expensive in that the social and family costs are high and that treatment of several kinds brought no important change.

SUMMARY

Hospital staff meet the patient and family at the point when the last 'holding group', usually the family, breaks down and a new group, therapeutic as provided by the hospital, is required by the patient and his 'holding group'. Everyone concerned had tried to handle his feelings about the disturbance by adjustments, more or less costly, such as reallocation of work and home roles, sometimes in entirety. Medical treatment is but one of these reallocations. It was a task undertaken with decreasing success by the family and is now handed over to the hospital. Many reallocations in the research sample were hard to measure as investments. Some, seen in retrospect at the time of the survey, had immense value; others seemed total losses inasmuch as they led neither to the reinstatement of the patient in the desired role nor to any new forms of social reconnection. *They seemed only to protect the community from becoming aware of the problem.* Estimating the gravity of the breakdown depended on:

(*a*) the nature of the special arrangements made
(*b*) how far these fitted personal norms of behaviour
(*c*) how long they could be maintained
(*d*) how far they were reversible.

The breakdown, at the point when the 'holding group' repudiated its task, was preceded by failure of relationships in other groups, notably at work and with friends. Rehabilitation reverses the process: aid from the natural emotional resources of non-medical people emerged as an important asset, difficult and expensive to manufacture synthetically as part of a national health service. Where family, work group, and friends remained attached to the patient, secondary breakdown was less likely. The patient was shown to be in a larger social network, contributing positively or negatively, and increasing the group's assets or liabilities. One important effect of treatment was the alteration in the pattern of membership of these groups.

Very early during the study we were faced with the inescapable fact that the method of assessment could never be precise and in no one case does it offer more than an approximation of actual costs. Moreover, the methods were essentially biased in terms of the individual and his family and ignored such factors as the cost of national insurance and the economics of industrial performance. But the study illustrated the limitations of simple financial or medical assessments based on the individual and ignoring one of the most important systems he has, that of a network of relationships. There are, then, three forms of transaction around the sick person: *money, obligation*, and *affection*. And affection that has insight can gear the other two to their most effective pitch.

PART III

Family-centred Nursing (1956–1966)

Editorial Note

An understanding in depth of the emotional development of the child, and of its reflection in adult behaviour and feeling, has always been the basis of nurse training in the hospital. Family-centred nursing was a natural and inevitable outcome.

T. F. Main remarks on the slow return of Western civilization to the practice of conserving the mother-child relationship during illness and hospitalization and links this to his own thinking, strongly influenced by his early teacher, Sir James Spence, and by the work of Spitz, Anna Freud, and Bowlby, which led to the gradual integration of mothers and children and, later, of complete families, into the hospital community.

His second paper, a penetrating dissertation on the phantasies of mothering, follows Doreen Weddell's account of the learning opportunities for nurses presented when families were admitted for treatment.

Four nurses describe their own experiences in developing the new facilities required in the hospital. Christine Schodt contributes a report on nursing a group of mothers and children, and describes the impact of these newcomers on the hospital. Joan Rush gives a personal account of her development of the nursery school. Doreen Martin describes her work with the adolescent group, a new and often turbulent ingredient in the life of the hospital. Janice Webster shows how the parents devised their own supportive techniques and, with their children, brought the hospital and the neighbourhood into closer contact.

Part III concludes with a paper by Hazel Edwards, indicating further developments in the hospital community and some later modifications in nurse training.

13 · *Mothers with Children on a Psychiatric Unit*[1]

BY T. F. MAIN

The current practice in Western hospitals of conserving mother-child relationships sprang from the lowliest origins – a near-slum in Newcastle-upon-Tyne, where, during the munitions drive in 1917, a day nursery had been created for the infants of mothers working in the factories. After the war the nursery continued to operate under voluntary support, and under medical aegis increasingly took over the care of ailing infants.

However, finances were limited, and even the bill for crockery breakages steadily worried its lay committee. Finally, they hit on a way of providing clean milk of perfect composition cheaply – and without using any crockery at all: the nursery employed unmarried mothers as maids and paid them 6*d.* a pint for their surplus milk. That this source of supply was not problem-free is shown by the records. For instance, Bessie, a ward maid, had to be dismissed when her yield dropped to 2 oz a day. But a new unique step – the provision of human milk for babies in Western clinics – had been taken.

By 1929 this nursery had become the Babies Hospital. Under the scientific stimulus of Dr (later Sir) J. C. Spence it began to encourage mothers to visit their sick babies regularly, to cuddle, nurse, and feed them; it provided accommodation for some to sleep there overnight. This innovation – the provision of mothers for children in hospital – arose primarily as a by-product of medical concern with the proper kind of milk for sick infants. However, Spence quickly realized that from this preservation of the mother-child relationship a bonus of hitherto unexpected and

[1] Reprinted from *Frontiers in General Hospital Psychiatry*, edited by L. Linn (New York: International Universities Press, 1961).

unrealized value for the lives and health of sick infants occurred. In 1942, in the full knowledge that infants do not live by milk alone, that important emotional issues are also involved in keeping mother and child together, forty-five mothers were admitted to the hospital. From then on, the staff became aware of the fact that the added physical and emotional complications attendant on separation were a vital aspect of the diseases of infancy, and must be given due consideration in treatment.

At first, only the benefits derived by the infants as a result of such practices were emphasized; the benefits to their mothers were little noticed. However, in a review of his programme, published in 1946, Spence stated:

> 'Each mother and child lived together in their own room arranged to give an atmosphere of domestic comfort which could not be alien to them. In the background there were experienced nurses and doctors to give technical aid when required. The mother was given as much responsibility as possible receiving, for example, her child straight from the operating theatre into her own arms. She lived with the child continually and at all stages shared fully in the credit for its recovery. A contrasting group of mothers, with infants similarly ill, remained at home while their infants were treated in hospital. They endured the usual anxiety of separation and waiting which is common to these circumstances, and which no man or woman who has not experienced it can appreciate. After a few weeks each mother returned to the hospital to receive her child at the hands of someone to whom she gave the credit for its care and cure. A study of these two groups of women over many years has revealed remarkable differences. In sharing experiences with their children, they first built up their confidences and enhanced their capacity. They returned to their homes and their neighbours with a sense of achievement which stood them in good stead afterwards. The other group had a sense of failure which reacted unfavourably on the child. They were obsessed by the dangers of trifling symptoms. A *necessary continuity of experience* had been broken, through being parted in those critical weeks of anxiety' (Spence, 1946; italics added).

From these small beginnings there has since been a steady growth in paediatric hospitals of practices designed to conserve the mother-child relationship, such as allowing mothers to visit frequently and at all hours, or to be admitted with their infants and toddlers. But it is indeed curious that these practices have taken so long to develop in the face of the evidence available for many years, produced first by paediatricians and later by psychiatrists, of the infant's needs for the mother, of the damage that can ensue from his separation from good mothering sources. The penalties of hospitalization of the infant were noted by Chapin as long ago as 1915, and subsequently by Lowrey (1940), Bender and Yarnell (1941), Bakwin (1942), Goldfarb (1943, 1944 a, b), Burlingham and Anna Freud (1944), Spitz (1945), and Bowlby (1946). Paediatricians, psychologists, and psychiatrists had, over a decade ago, contributed significant observations on the serious effects of infant-rearing without adequate mothering. Certainly, one must wonder why the social application of their findings has been negligible to date.

It is also curious that little or no attention has been paid to the effects of separation, if it is the mother who is admitted to a hospital because of illness. In Western countries she is usually cut off from all contact with her children, whether she wants it or not, and her child is bereft of her; moreover, ideas of her illness and death may permeate the child's environment more than ever. Yet, in most hospitals it is not thought proper for children, especially young children, to visit their sick mothers. The reasons vary: a sick mother should not be bothered by children; children increase the risk of infections in a hospital; they may be noisy and disturb the other patients. Such reasons are, of course, partially based on the truth that children can be a nuisance; but others are based on an incorrect hypothesis that the children will be harmed by such contact.

No one would deny that for many situations these arguments are valid; but when applied to all hospitals they recall the hostile ratiocinations common a few years ago when it was first generally mooted that the child in a hospital should have frequent visits from his mother. These arguments underestimated the importance of the child's relationship with his mother to his mental and physical health.

It is even more curious that, in view of the scientific and practical concern given to disruption of the mother-child pair, the psychological problems of the child should receive almost exclusive emphasis and those of the mother so little. It is as though we have forgotten that mothering is a feat of feminine maturity often precariously arrived at, and that the brittle mothering capacity of some women can be damaged beyond recovery through separation from their infants, leaving the mother-child relationship thereafter beset by mutual dissonance. Even in this matter I would draw attention to the temptation to regard such an outcome as a tragedy only for the infant, and not for the mother as well.

These somewhat petulant words are directed first to myself and are the result of hindsight. In 1948, when a woman referred to the Cassel Hospital (for the inpatient treatment of severe neurosis) asked if she could bring her toddler son with her, since there was no one else to care for him, I was interested in the penalties of separating mother and child as they related, first, to the child's physical and emotional health, and, second, and hardly at all, to the woman's confidence in her future capacities as a mother. It may have been the memory of my student days with Spence, as well as my interest in the work of René Spitz in New York, and of Anna Freud and John Bowlby in London, that made me agree to the woman's request. In any event, what began as an unusual, occasional occurrence has since come to be a common and unremarkable element of the programme of this psychiatric hospital for adults, until today it is the rule for a mother seeking admission to bring her young children with her, even though at first glance she may seem to be too crippled by emotional illness to care for them. However, this programme had a slow development. Perhaps it had to be slow, to allow ample time for staff attitudes to change, and to permit growth of procedures.

During the first six years of this experiment the hospital staff was occupied with the study of something of more importance to it than the problems of mother and child in a hospital, although it included consideration of these problems. The project under way at that time is highly relevant, however, to the development of our present procedures, and must therefore be described.

THE HOSPITAL COMMUNITY AS A BACKGROUND TO TREATMENT

We had become aware that the view of a hospital as a place which can best treat severely ill patients because it houses a co-ordinated concentrate of various technical procedures was incomplete. We were also aware that patients admitted to the hospital for 'treatment' were thereby – in addition and almost by accident – encouraged to assume social roles and relations of a distinct, but so far as we were concerned, unstudied kind. These may be summarized, without undue distortion, in such terms as powerless, irresponsible, invalid, regressed, conforming. We began to question the assumption that roles and relations of this regressed sort, so necessary for patients with acute bodily illness, were also appropriate for psychiatric illness, where regression is a basic issue.

Clinical experience had shown us that the hospital's alloplastic responses to a patient's distress were sometimes in contrast to the aims of treatment, that is, that he undertake autoplastic changes; and that the relationships offered to a patient in the hospital were sometimes not merely incidental to, but decisive for, the success or failure of therapy. The relationships established between patients and staff were, of course, partly the result of patient expectations, but also much the result of traditional hospital staff training in 'proper' medical, nursing, and domestic roles.

We reviewed these matters critically and thereafter set out to study continuously and to experiment with the hospital's staff and patient roles, relations, and structures.[1] Our aim was to create a community in which patients would not automatically have to disrupt so many of their ordinary and important relationships, where they would not have to surrender their initiative and responsibility for deciding on the thousand and one details of their daily lives. These experiments queried the covert, but commonly held, assumptions that the role of the patient in a hospital is to be ill, disturbed, grateful, quiet, powerless, and in need of a staff which is omniscient, selfless, powerful, and firm.[2]

We offered the patients, individually and collectively, many of the powers and responsibilities, hitherto held by the staff, for making or carrying out those decisions by which the daily life of the patient is ordered. The staff also participated in the growth of new concepts of the hospital's purpose, in many revisions of their own roles, relations, and structure. Indeed, these changes had to occur *pari passu* with changes in the patients' community. The staff had to undergo attitude changes in such elementary matters as the common hospital ethos that 'the staff knows best' (and senior staff better than junior), as well as more touchy issues, for example, that nurses have feelings which are not always creditable. Meanwhile, there was a danger to be watched for – that halting the retreat

[1] See Chapters 4, 5, and 6 – Ed.
[2] See Chapter 1 – Ed.

by patients and staff from the realities of everyday life might result in a different kind of tyranny – the denial of the right to be ill. We had to tolerate psychological disturbance and treat it by psychoanalysis and psychotherapy, and, at the same time, make the hospital less of a social vacuum. We sought to make it a place which could tolerate experimentation, and mistakes, and offer opportunities for the pleasures of stress as well as of relaxation, and we tried to fashion these efforts on the patterns of the ordinary lives to which all patients eventually belong.

During these developments, both clinical and sociological experience, sometimes dearly bought, had shown us that the desocialization of a patient in a psychiatric hospital is neither wise nor necessary. We knew the peril of submitting patients to heavy external strain, but we also knew the peril of attempting to protect them from all strain, and we were seeking a system that would provide strains optimal[1] for therapy.

We wanted to provide only such support as was necessary. Living in the hospital community presented obligations and realistically based tasks, and the strains derived therefrom. But the hospital was also capable of elastic adaptation to the capacities of individual members. Eventually, it became normal (though not universal) for patients to work at their ordinary jobs while in the hospital. Some patients worked at jobs outside the hospital; housewives took on similar working roles, housekeeping in the hospital.

MOTHERS IN HOSPITALS

Thus we became aware of the fact that to hospitalize a mother and separate her from her children was unwittingly to compel a divorce from *her* job of mothering, and from the children who made it. For the sake of aiding the mothers' treatment alone, women were therefore increasingly permitted to bring their young children on admission. We had learned of the advantages to the children in such a procedure, and we knew it was a doubtful investment in mental hygiene to treat mothers, but ignore their children's needs. Now, however, we put the accent on the benefits to the mother, and tentatively feel our way forward case by case.

[1] I confess that this word optimal is imprecise, but I cannot improve on it. At best I can say it lies somewhere between maximal and minimal.

Thus up to 1954 we had made no special study of mothers or of mothering. Rather, we had seen ourselves as treating women patients; the admission of their children was simply an unusual feature of their stay, requested by them and agreed to by us, and part of our general attempt to keep patients in touch with their ordinary life. The neuroses of these mothers had centred particularly on the mother-child relationship. Nevertheless, we learned from them.

We noticed that admitting the pair certainly helped to maintain and promote the positive elements in the mother-child relationship, but also that it prevented escape from and concealment of negative elements. Increasing experience had led us to suspect that admitting a mother by herself was sometimes to collude with her hostility towards her children, or at least with her wish to be separated from them, and this was confirmed when we now began to inquire further into the cases of those mothers who requested solitary admission, and actively to invite all mothers to bring their children. Not all welcomed our invitation; some were afraid of it. Bringing the children of unwilling mothers into the hospital pointed up for us and their mothers their difficulties in daily living, often as a matter for urgent treatment. These difficulties would have been hidden from us all (for the mothers sometimes had scotomata for them) had we admitted the mothers alone.

From 1955 on, we made it a condition of admission that mothers bring their babies and young children with them. Few exceptions have been necessary, and these have concerned mothers whose terror of association with the child or inability to care for him has been overwhelming. Even in these cases the mother has requested the admission of the child within a week or two; and we are of the opinion that such requests occur too early to be attributed to therapy. Rather, the experience of being in a hospital community which contains other mothers and their babies has been sufficient to encourage these women to make another attempt at motherhood.

The mothers and children thus enter a hospital where other patients are already engaged in fairly active roles as a matter of course. They see childless patients leaving the hospital daily to carry out full-time or part-time paid or unpaid work. Earlier generations of patients have made it commonplace not to abandon pre-admission interests or responsibilities, and in this culture it is commonplace for baby care to take its place among the other domestic activities of patients who help each other to cook or wash dishes, make beds, darn socks, sew curtains, decorate rooms, shop for hospital groceries, plan the hospital menus, etc. The patients have come to regard such jobs as being within their scope. These are ordinary chores needed by the community, often a nuisance; but they carry with them their own reality and rewards in functional relations with others. And it is unremarkable for new patients, sometimes expecting invalid roles, to become active in these matters at a rate which surprises their doctors and relatives.

On the other hand, the hospital offers some security. If work is commonplace, so is illness. Fellow patients and staff can accept and provide for individual distress, anxiety, depression, rages, etc., with discernment within patient-created social mores and discipline. This is not an unplanned society, and the nursing staff has by now a considerable sophistication at diagnosing and intervening in the hidden social conflicts that are now known to be so productive of individual tension; at helping patients to find ways of solving daily living problems; and at relating fairly optimally and without compulsiveness to distressed patients. The standards of child care are decided by the mothers and their right to bring up their children in their own ways is respected, even if it is not approved. While there is no one to absolve any mother from final responsibility for her child, the community around her is ready to accept the difficulties she may have in discharging this responsibility, and to regard these with sympathy and practical help, individually or collectively. Patients may provide for her special needs, and share her chores of child-rearing, and in any crisis she is likely to get not censure but inquiry and support from those around her.

She will find other mothers who know something of the emotional disturbances consequent on mothering, who will help her to maintain her domestic and mothering skills. This group effect in a responsible self-disciplining community is not easy to describe, but the help of recovering mothers often has an earthy sanity which is a vital part of the nursing potential of the hospital. The mothers do not expect perfection of each other, for all know that mothering contains stresses, that children can be annoying. When one mother fell ill physically and heard that she had to go to a surgical hospital within the hour, without her baby, another mother, who four months ago had been quite intolerant of her own child, volunteered to look after the sick mother's as well as her own. Not all forms of help are as obvious as this, but the cumulative effect of many smaller incidents in providing security is considerable.

The community effect is important in altering behaviour, in maintaining or avoiding unnecessary regression, but it is not, of course, decisive for psychotherapy. Each mother has regular sessions with her psychotherapist, and it is these that finally determine fundamental change.

The hospital has a hundred beds, placed in some twenty single rooms and in other rooms with two, three, four, five, and six beds – and the whole hospital is easily arranged into four units of approximately equal size, each self-contained, with twenty-five beds per unit, and its own kitchen, bathrooms, washing and drying facilities, all at the disposal of patients without staff supervision. Each of these four units (or medical firms) has its own medical and nursing staff. Each firm, under a consultant, is entirely responsible for its own area and its own affairs, for its own domestic and nursing arrangements and its own methods of treatment.

The maintenance, repairs, and redecoration, the daily cleaning of the area, are the responsibility of the firm; and the daily work cannot be carried on without the help of the patients, who are largely responsible to themselves and to each other for deciding what is needed, what gets done domestically, and who does it. Each firm has a small annual budget which it is free to spend on internal decoration, curtain material, washing and drying arrangements, and so on. The patients in a firm meet with the sisters weekly to discuss what shall be done, and by whom, and invariably the discussions include recognition of the particular liabilities or assets, critical needs or trustworthy potential, of the various patients in the firm.

In this setting the problems created by patients (including mothers and children) and their special requirements can be formally discussed weekly by them and by others, and appropriate arrangements are made. Both patients and staff are aware that the resources of each firm in money, accommodation, and labour are limited, and that the solution of such everyday issues as the need for quiet when a baby is sleeping, for a laundry and ironing services, or for the repair of furniture is a matter for decision by and co-operation from all. These weekly meetings set a climate in which individual and communal problems can be openly recognized and discussed, and in which patients can be exposed to the criticism of others and can offer to help each other. Anxious mothers can get the support of others, and when a mother is felt to be neglecting her baby both nurses and patients can plan to help. The friendships between patients and the ventures on which they embark together do much to compensate for the corporate discipline that they demand of each other, rather as in a family. At these meetings there is fairly honest give and take over the solution of practical issues, beset though these might be by emotional problems.

The hospital also has central administrative services, common rooms, dining room, workshops, and entertainment rooms, and a patients' central organization decides the appropriate codes of behaviour in these areas. Each firm is responsible for providing some general service in these central areas, such as food preparation or washing up, cleaning and maintaining common rooms and other areas. The patients' central organization has arranged that mothers and children should have special meal-times so that the nuisance of noise, jammy fingers, and spilt milk is shared only by mothers and not by other patients, that toys and disorder should be confined to *one* of the common rooms, that guards and railings are erected as necessary, that extra milk should be available for children, that the children's television hours should be sacred for them, and so on.

Each mother and child live together in their own room, 'arranged to give an atmosphere of domestic comfort' and even homely disorder 'which could not be alien to them', and to which the mother brings the child's own cot, linen, and toys from home. There is a perambulator park near the hospital entrance. With or without help from others the mother cares for her child, launders for him, prepares his food in the ward kitchen, and nurses him. Every morning sees mothers pushing their children in prams in the local shopping centre, or washing and hanging out laundry in the hospital grounds with their children 'put out' in prams or running beside them, or playing with others. Meal-times see mothers feeding babies on their knees or in their own high chairs with hospital adult food, or with milk meals they have prepared themselves. Afternoons may see the children playing in gangs in the hospital or the grounds while their mothers are busy elsewhere; or a mother may be soothing her infant to sleep in a darkened room, or nursing him in the garden. Evenings may see the fathers of these children as familiar visitors eating at the hospital with their wives and helping with the washing up afterwards, handling, potting, or bathing the baby, and thereafter joining their wives over games or television or taking them to a nearby cinema. Weekends may see husbands in slippers staying the night with their wives as lodgers in the hospital, or some mothers and children spending nights at home so that they can cook the family Sunday dinner and see the older children.

It is remarkable how many mothers, who in a more orthodox hospital context would be very ill, passive, and dependent, are able to carry on fairly actively, supported by each other and by their psychotherapy. The hospital tries to possess neither mother nor child, but to offer independence and to provide support only when it is necessary; to be, in other words, the agent of the home and family rather than to replace these as the centre of the patient's life.

Although we continue to admit mothers with general neurotic problems with their children, we have increasingly had referred to us severe neurotic problems overtly centring on the mother-child relationship. These are roughly of two kinds. First, they have included puerperal upsets where the advent of the child has precipitated acute illnesses: depression, with apathy towards the baby; anxiety states, with hatred of him; infanticidal wishes; amnesias for the birth or the baby's daily whereabouts, or fearful neglect; and ambulant schizophrenia with disturbed relations to all, including perhaps the baby.[1] Second, we have admitted mothers whose relationship with the baby has deteriorated from an initial good start until at the toddler age mothering is fraught with anxieties, rages, murderous wishes, or hysterical symptoms. The most disturbed of these mothers have given us anxious moments – where it would have been tempting to forget the whole problem by separating the pair or recommending adoption – but the whole community has slowly grown in confidence in its capacity to help these women, and we have come to count on an improvement occurring within ten days of admission up to a point where the relationship becomes tolerable to the mother and those around her.

[1] Women with puerperal confusional insanity or schizophrenia of certifiable extent are not admitted.

This rewarding improvement certainly cannot be attributed to specific psychotherapy, but rather to the effects of joint hospitalization. My colleague, Peter Lomas, has described the modification of guilt over becoming a mother as a result of the hospital's many implicit sanctions, and the expiation of guilt by the 'disgrace' of having to confess failure and being admitted to the hospital (Lomas, 1959, 1960). We would add that hospital life reduces the demands on the patient's ego during a time when it is under maximal stress from the outer and inner worlds for various reasons not to be discussed here. However, the empiric fact is that these improvements do occur.

NURSING AND ADMISSION PROBLEMS

The nurses' tasks with mothers have involved special problems of training. The nursing techniques have been, in general, to avoid advising, instructing, or deciding for patients, but to be on hand as co-workers and discussants when the patients wish to discuss their difficulties before making decisions of their own; and to intervene in group crises which patients create for themselves and each other. This is a difficult nursing technique to apply, and especially difficult with those patients who have a great capacity to arouse guilt, pity, or omnipotence in others. In such circumstances a nurse may be sorely tempted to treat a patient like a child and to think and decide for her in ways which, whatever their useful short-term results, tend to blur the patient's ego autonomy and create addicted dependency and helplessness.

It is particularly difficult for the nursing staff to remain both sympathetic and objective with distressed mothers. Some mothers are piteous in their concern for the very child they might be savagely neglecting or wishing to harm. Others who pursue a policy of guilt-driven dangerous permissiveness or cold repressiveness equally tempt the nurse to impulsive, unobjective responses. The distress of the infants and toddlers in the care of such mothers is an added nursing strain, and frequently the nurses (like the other members of the hospital population, including the administrative staff) have felt tempted to take over the care of these children. Childless spinsters themselves, some nurses may have very personal reasons for welcoming the advent of children to whom they might become important, and for resenting their inefficient mothers. When the mother herself is only too glad to hand the care of her child over to another, the temptation is even greater.

Only the slow working through of these matters in nurses' discussion groups has permitted them to maintain their own nursing techniques, to hold together the mother-child unit, and to nurse its stresses while according full eventual responsibility to the mother. The very recognition by the nurses of the temptations around them has become part of the accepted nursing skills, and the reward is considerable. There is a deep satisfaction in aiding a mother's recovery – if only for the sake of the child.

Mothers and children are admitted, as is common procedure, on request from their family doctors, child guidance clinics, psychiatrists, or mother and child welfare clinics. We have found that a home visit by a senior nursing sister who is later to care for the pair in the hospital, and full consideration of her findings at a preliminary case conference, are helpful in anticipating future nursing problems and in deciding whether the mother should be admitted with more than one child, how far the husband should be brought into the treatment situation, etc. During her home visit the nurse tells the family what they should bring in the way of high chair, cot, pram, toys, and so forth; she makes plain from the first, by suggesting frequent visiting of wife by family, and family by wife, that admission to the hospital does not imply the possession of a family member by strangers, but rather the offer of treatment within continued family relationships.

A curious difficulty frequently arises in puerperal cases, with regard to these home visits. Though the home visit is made immediately after the request for admission, it frequently happens that the family cannot be found at its home address! Puerperal breakdown is sometimes an explosive family catastrophe involving great panic, concern, or anger. The sick mother may have fled to the protection of a female relative; the father may be with neighbours or his family of origin; the baby may be in the care of additional relatives, neighbours, or a child-care home. The job of the visiting nurse is now to pick up the family pieces and to expedite admission. This is not easy, for feelings run high, and the offer to the mother of reunion with her baby may be strongly resisted. Maternity is very much a family affair, and the handling of family tensions by solutions which are mutually arrived at is our aim. The husband cannot be excluded from the original arrangements, and the nurse must handle the mother's initial fears of being bullied, separated from her baby, or forced to be with him. The admission of puerperal breakdowns is a matter of some emergency, and requires social skill.

We have admitted up to three children with one mother, and occasionally we have had to arrange school classes for older children, but it is more usual for a mother to bring only one toddler or infant. Thus she may be nursed in a single room with space for a cot, as mentioned earlier, or in a double room when there is more than one child. Rarely, where the father too has been psychologically ill, we have admitted whole families and have used two rooms. Where a mother and child must share a room with another patient, a childless patient seems a more desirable solution than another mother-child pair, and this seems to be no greater hardship for the childless patient. Occasionally, we have housed a child in a different room from his mother, but this is rare. Our doubts about the wisdom of having toddlers sleep in the same rooms as their mothers are the less, because such arrangements with disturbed children or mothers are almost the rule in their own homes.

The hospital is not mainly concerned with mothers and children, and there is no exclusive unit for them. They live as ordinary a life as possible, cheek by jowl with other patients, but they tend to congregate together. There are usually fifteen to thirty-five children in the hospital at any one time, and because the mothers bring their own equipment and conduct their own baby care, the average cost for maintaining each young child is low – some £2. 5*s.* per week – but it is much higher for the occasional older children who occupy an adult hospital bed and eat full hospital meals. It must be remarked, in this connection, that substantial economies in nursing care are effected by allowing patients in the hospital to take active roles in management.

None of the psychiatric staff has felt confident regarding children's physical upsets and infectious diseases, and the hospital has enlisted the help of Dr C. A. Baggley, our local general practitioner, on whose panel the children are registered, and who visits them in the hospital unless their mothers are able to take them to his surgery. The mothers themselves have instituted regular visits to the local maternity and child welfare clinic which they attend in small groups. We have drawn freely on the generous advice of Dr Eric Pereira, the medical officer of health for Richmond, in dealing with outbreaks of infectious disease.

THE EFFECT OF THE PROGRAMME ON OTHER PATIENTS

In the early days both mothers and children met with complex emotional reactions from the other more or less seriously disturbed adult patients, whose own miseries and regressed needs led to an ambivalent warmth about these sick mothers and children. Some patients felt deposed and displaced, with the babies as their rivals for the attention of the staff; others argued that the hospital was bad for children because of the neurotic behaviour of the rest of the community; still others said that their cure was jeopardized because it depended on peace and quiet, now endangered by the new arrivals. Some patients, again, spoke on behalf of the mothers, whose illness, they claimed, was due to the demands made on them by their offspring. The patients' attitudes, expressed in the minutes of their firm meetings and of their central committee, veered between the one extreme that children were dangerous intruders, who should be kept in special departments, well disciplined, and not allowed to mix with adults, and the other extreme that their noise and disorder should at all times be tolerated.

With the working through of these attitudes, sensible arrangements were made of a fairly ordinary domestic kind. By the summer of 1955, men patients had erected swings for the children, made tables for the boilers, and helped to arrange drying racks, clothes horses, clothes lines, and blackboards. But when cold weather drove the children indoors, emotional extremes could again be noticed. The patients' executive committee considered compulsory quiet periods, a special unit for mothers and children, a noise room with a rota of mothers to supervise it, and excluding children from the television rooms – as well as, on the other hand, creating special programmes and privileges for them which ignored the rights of adults. Ultimately, few of these recommendations survived.

With the passage of time, mothers and children have ceased to become special, and strong emotional attitudes towards them, either tough or sentimental, have vanished. Washing, drying, and eating arrangements, one common room for children's toys and apparatus, and arrangements for mothers to keep in touch with their own homes, have become routine. Issues that a year ago were hot have now cooled.

But though, for patients and staff alike, settlement of the affairs of mothers and children has become part of the daily work of the hospital, this work is not, and cannot be, effortless. Staff and patients continue to be confronted with problems of feeling and behaviour, manifested as relatively trivial practical issues, whose solution has not been easy.

THE EFFECT OF THE PROGRAMME ON THE CHILDREN

Initially, we had fears for the emotional welfare of young children cared for by seriously neurotic mothers in a community of other neurotic patients. These were the greater because the children were known to have been under emotional distress because of disturbance in their mothers, and after admission their own behaviour disturbances were apparent. On the other hand, they were attached to their mothers and all but a few have benefited indirectly, but quickly, from improvements in their mothers' attitudes. Nor have we found other patients disturbing to the children. Neurotic patients' difficulties lie mostly in relation to other adults and rarely preclude the ordinary ambivalent altruistic responses which young children evoke in most people. They have no close or intimate contact with the children unless they wish it, for the children belong to their mothers and live and play in their vicinity and with each other. I know of only one adult patient who was refused admission out of consideration for mothers and children – a man with homicidal impulses towards children; and I am not sure from my experiences of mothers with similar impulses that even here the decision was necessary or wise.

My colleague, the late Imre Gluck, much concerned himself with the group treatment of mothers of toddlers and steadily correlated his findings with the observations of the hospital psychologists, M. Wrenn and E. H. Rayner, who have studied the children's behaviour in group play sessions. (Gluck and Wrenn, 1959). These workers have made precise observations which confirm the general impression stated above that children in the hospital benefit indirectly but quickly from improvements in their mothers' attitudes. It is fair to say that children flourish in the hospital, and, whatever the disadvantages, these are distinctly fewer than would be evoked by lengthy separation and later reunion.

It may well be, however, that this manner of handling psychiatric disturbances in mothers contains subtle snags. Follow-up by letter indicates that the mother-child relationship is not disturbed when the pair return home and that the children settle down quickly and unremarkably alongside their mothers in their homes. However, older children may miss the hospital and their companions there for some days after they return. It has been well said that, for a baby, home is simply where the mother is, but more adequate follow-up visits may reveal hidden problems of resettlement with older children of which we are as yet unaware.

CONCLUSIONS

Because we do not admit chronic cases, or those under certificate, we have no experiences with grossly psychotic mothers and their children. Nor are we sure that our procedure could suitably be used for all disturbed mothers. Some of our patients needed psychotherapy before their anxieties were lowered sufficiently for them to agree that their children should accompany them; and sooner or later we shall meet cases (say, of autistic mothers) in which the child would be better separated from the mother than made to coexist with her. But we have been impressed by how much can be achieved with these women. Some of our mothers had been certified in the recent past, and many had been in mental hospitals. Some had found mothering an impossible task, and either they or their husbands had sought foster parents for their infants. In the hospital, severely disturbed, terrified, depressed, or impulse-ridden women become able to mother their children with increasing mutual benefit, and eventually to help other mothers and children.

I would add that psychiatry needs opportunities to study severe disturbances of the mother-child relationship, for it is to be expected that study of the gross disturbances will reveal these to be but exaggerations of the much more common, almost universal, minor disturbances. A great deal of the literature deals with the psychology of women, and also of infants, but remarkably little has been written on mothering and its disturbances; and most of what has been written is concerned with the baby's needs rather than the mother's. Since it is in the area of mothering that preventive psychiatry is likely to make its best investment, this is indeed surprising. Perhaps it is partly because it is our usual practice to separate mother and child, when there is an acute disturbance of mothering, that we have been denied opportunities for extending our knowledge in this obviously important field. Admitting mothers and children to psychiatric hospitals may therefore be an important development for research as well as treatment.

14 · *Family-centred Nursing*[1]

BY DOREEN WEDDELL

In spite of the work carried out in recent years by psycho-analysts, anthropologists, and sociologists in elucidating the interrelationships of the family as they are seen in the psychic life of the individual, between members of a family, and between the family and society, the nurse in hospital has remained surprisingly guarded and suspicious in her relationship with the family of her patient. Even children's nurses tended to feel that parents were a necessary but often an irritating adjunct to a child's admission to hospital. Only in recent years have they been able to recognize that the child's tie with his mother is to be cherished rather than interfered with or broken. For nurses in a general hospital ward, the patient's family is still often felt only as an added burden with which they have to deal as best they can, rather than as an essential part of a distressed situation that they must nurse. To psychiatric nurses, the family of the long-stay patient may often hardly exist, and the hospital maternity nurse's need to possess mother and baby is well known. Visiting times are too often felt by nurses as just part of the routine, an unwanted intrusion, and are not always arranged to suit the needs of the patient and family. There seem to be few hospitals where the nursing task is shared with the family as members of the nursing team.

The nurses' interest in working with the family at the Cassel Hospital grew from their psychological understanding of an infant's, child's, and adult's need of his family, rather than from any sentimentality or imposed procedures. The nurse's perception of her role, and the procedures derived from it, were already based

[1] Paper read at the Panel on Psychiatric Nursing, Third World Congress of Psychiatry, Montreal, 1961, and published in the *International Nursing-Review*, Vol. 8, No. 6, 1961.

on the formulation that she seeks to achieve a relationship in which the healthy part of the patient can be worked with and respected. Spitz's film, *Grief* (1946), and the work of Dorothy Burlingham and Anna Freud (1942, 1944) and of Bowlby (1946), directed the nurse's attention to what might be happening to the children of mothers who were patients in the hospital. Melanie Klein's analysis of very young children (1932), which demonstrated the possibility of understanding a child's feelings, phantasies, and internal and external relationships as revealed in play, helped the nurse further to recognize the reality of the patient's psychic life. Working with children in a day nursery, as part of her training, gave the nurse opportunity to link theory with practice and facilitated her understanding of the child still present in herself and in her patients. Winnicott's idea that there is no such thing as an infant, that there can be only an *infant-mother* unit which, if it is to function satisfactorily, needs the father's *hold*-support of his wife as she *hold*-supports the child, showed the nurse that on occasion her role would be to *hold*-support the family.[1] Her role with the mothers who brought their children into hospital would be to help them to continue to care for their families as they did at home.

The husband accompanies his wife and children to hospital and is encouraged to visit whenever he can, to help to put the children to bed, and, perhaps, to take his wife out for the evening. He may come in as a patient himself. Sometimes the husband tries to get the nurse to give him 'psychological treatment'. She, however, tries not to get involved as the exclusive confidant of either the wife or the husband but will see them together, interfering as little as possible with the normal family situation, but available in any difficulty. When husband and wife fight, one walking out fed up with the other, the nurse will talk over the trouble with them. Sometimes other patients will act as arbitrators; the therapist may discuss the matter in a treatment session but, as a general rule, he will not be involved during the actual disturbance. The nurses also discuss any areas of disagreement among themselves which may be reflected in the patients' disagreement.

The nurse, will, of course, be interested in the children's development and the effect of coming into hospital. A child often reflects the mother's anxiety and the nurse sees it as her role not to do anything with or for the child herself but to deal with the mother's

[1] See also Chapter 19 – Ed.

problem. She will try to understand the difficulty the mother may be having with the child, her husband, another patient, her therapist, or with the nurse herself. She will not necessarily do anything more than verbalize what she thinks the mother is feeling, so helping her to maintain her relationships in the external world while the therapist and the mother investigate the upset in her inner world.

The children will miss their fathers if they cannot see them as often as they do at home. Sometimes, if the father is not around very much, they will make a kind of uncle of other men, staff or patients.

Two kinds of nursing relationship can be identified: first, with families in which the mother was ill before marriage and whose illness now disturbs the whole family, and, second, with families in which the mother becomes ill as a result of some specific event, such as childbirth, as the following examples will show.

One week-end a mother was certain that her child, Nancy, aged three, was ill. The local doctor must be called at once. The nurse knew that the husband was not coming this week-end. Nancy sometimes went home to her father when he did not come to the hospital. The patient was pregnant and did not want the child. So the nurse had to think: Is it the wife's anxiety about her husband not coming, or a transference reaction to her therapist being away? (As a general rule, no treatment sessions are given at the week-ends.) Is the child distressed about not seeing her father, or is there really an infection? The mother was sure Nancy had a lump behind her ear. True, she had a slightly raised temperature, was fretful and unhappy, and nothing seemed to satisfy her. The nurse called in the local doctor as the mother wished, not because she felt anxious herself but because she felt he could be something of a substitute for the absent husband and therapist for the patient, and a father figure for the child. No treatment was prescribed and the next day both patient and child were better. Nancy, however, was later seen sitting in a chair pressing a big red ball to her tummy, talking to it, patting it, and throwing it away. Her anxiety about her mother's pregnancy was made clear by the play. It also turned out that the mother had been much concerned at the time with ideas of having the coming baby adopted.

If this incident had not happened at a week-end, the nurse might have tried to help the mother to contain her anxiety until the treatment session. One of the nursing skills lies in maintaining a friendly concern for the patient without becoming a readily available substitute for the therapist. This situation can be further complicated by the needs of the child in his own right, his ways of dealing with his mother as well as the use she may be making of him.

For those patients whose illness is the result of a particular event – childbirth – the nurse's role is somewhat different. With this illness, the family fragments rapidly. By the time the referring doctor's letter has reached the hospital and the nurse has arrived at the patient's home, the family is often already split up: father gone to his parents, mother to her mother, and the children to someone else, often the local welfare agency. The nurse's first task is to join the family up again in order to discuss the prospect of admission and the offer of treatment. Not only is the husband needed in the therapeutic team, he may become the chief source of nursing care. Here, the nurse's task is to support and reassure him in a role which, while it may bring satisfaction and relieve some of his jealousy of his wife's mothering capacity, may arouse guilt in so far as he feels he is usurping a role usually assigned to women.

To illustrate: one evening a call came from the local maternity hospital. Could we admit a patient, seven days *post partum*, very depressed and confused? The nurse went to the hospital, saw a very regressed patient who could hardly do anything for herself and needed her husband there all the time. After some difficulty, he agreed to take two weeks from work and come into hospital with his wife. During the next few days he virtually became a mother to her while she behaved like a baby, clinging to him, having to be fed and washed. Yet with the husband's support, who in turn was supported by the nurse, this very ill woman managed to suckle her baby and look after him. Meanwhile, in her therapeutic sessions, her confusion about herself and her baby was examined. Gradually she became less dependent on her husband and he could return to work and she to her home.

It is important for the nurse to understand how she may be experienced by these patients, some of whose difficulties arise from their having internalized an envious mother who, in the patient's phantasy, will hate her, may even kill her, if she becomes a mother herself. The patient feels she must placate this internal mother through suffering instead of enjoying her motherhood. She may even have to fail in her mothering for the same reason. It is obvious that the nurse, if she herself is unmarried, will envy the patient's childbearing capacity and may be led into a collusion with the patient to the extent of their agreeing together that the child would be better in other hands. The patient's wish to rid herself of the ties of motherhood, to have no husband and be single again, can sometimes lead to a useful discussion between the nurse and patient of their envy of each other.

Patients who may not be so disoriented as the above two examples nevertheless have destructive impulses and phantasies about their children. They present a different problem to the nurse. Her task here is to help them to nurse each other. In practice, there is often a good deal of mutual support and co-operation between patients. They will look after each other's children. The husbands may get together and redecorate a room or mend the children's toys.

We often see a dramatic change in patients on admission, before psychotherapy as such has begun. A young woman who a few hours before could not contemplate holding her baby, let alone feeding him or bathing him, will find herself doing just those things. She will be just as frightened as before, that she will drown the baby, or poison him, drop him or throw him out of the window; but she sees the other mothers who have the same fears looking after their babies, so, with their support, and that of her husband and the nurse, she tries her hand too. The nurse will usually be in the bathroom at bath-time if the patient feels safer that way; she may help the mother but will not, as a rule, do the bathing for her. Similarly, the nurse will sit with the mother while she is feeding the baby, if the mother wants her to. At night, when the mother is alone and anxious about her destructive impulses, it is usual for another patient to share a room with her. Again, other patients may look after the child along with their own if the mother is having a specially bad day. These arrangements will be discussed at meetings with the nursing staff. A particularly disturbed new patient often finds it helpful to share her fears with other patients and the nurses. Any difficulties she may have are then known by the others and the anxieties seem to be lessened.

Being with the mother and baby, listening and observing, will help the nurse to understand what the baby may mean to the mother. When the baby is fretful and difficult to satisfy, aggressive, scratching and biting his mother, and she feels she cannot stand him another minute, it is easy for the nurse to see that the baby is felt as the greedy, destructive part of the mother herself, which she cannot stand, or as the part of her husband which the wife is disappointed in and wishes to punish. The baby may be seen as a doll which the mother feels she can do as she likes with; or he may be a messy thing that has come out of her body, which she cannot bring herself to love and comfort. This understanding helps the nurse to assess the risk to the child from the mother's destructive impulses, and the risk to the mother from her suicidal wishes.

The mothers' capacity to tolerate and understand such impulses in each other has proved to be an important factor in the nursing technique. With their therapists, the patients gain some understanding of the sources of these fears and impulses; in discussion and activity with the nurses and each other, they feel less outcast. Nursing of this kind, however, is not easy to establish or to maintain. It makes great demands on the nurses and the therapists. They gain support by sharing, in meetings of various kinds, the anxiety that such patients arouse in them. The nurse, through recognizing some of the sources of her own love, hate, rivalry, and destructive, possessive, and restorative impulses, can understand to some extent what the patient is feeling and may thus be able to respond appropriately.

In countries less developed (so-called) than those of the West, a thesis describing a nurse's role such as this would be unnecessary and irrelevant. No one would go to hospital unless a close member of the family could go with him. Many factors, psychological, sociological, and physical, have led to the situation that, in Western countries, a sick member is almost dispossessed of his family on entering hospital. It may well be that continuing study of individual psychic experiences will clarify further the role of the family in health as well as in illness.

15 · *A Fragment on Mothering*[1]

BY T. F. MAIN

Mothering is a subject, like courting or dying, of personal concern to all mankind, carrying a high degree of emotional loading. Objective scientific observations and concepts about it are rare, whereas subjective views, either openly emotional or disguised under masses of rationalization, are common. It is not hard to find a reason for this: we were all once babies and we therefore knew, with a certainty born of personal passions and appetites, exactly how a mother ought to be. In our yells of delight or rage we began almost at once to express our views about mothering and now that we have the power of words we can preach, with an authority born of long personal experience of upbringing, about what makes a good mother. Mothers, for this reason as well as for others, rarely lack advisers, and it is interesting to note that most scientific studies about mothers and children are usually framed so that the child's psychology is put in the forefront and the child's needs are felt to be paramount. Even when the mother *is* studied or offered treatment there is sometimes the implication that this is less for her own sake than for her child's. We who are grown-up children tend to use a frame of reference in which she is the background of the child's life; it is uncommon for her to be taken as the initial figure for study, with the child as merely part of *her* background.

What mothering means to the child is certainly an important scientific question, meet to be pursued; but it is also important for science that we should grant equal attention to the question of what mothering means to mothers and study their behaviour not for the child's sake only, nor only to throw light on problems of infancy, but that we may learn something of maternal parenthood

[1] Reprinted from the *Davidson Clinic Bulletin*, Edinburgh, 1958.

as a step in the psychological development of women. It is plainly a difficult step, one that many otherwise fairly mature women shy at, with a host of reasons that sound better than they are, and one that many fail at in minor or major ways.

IDEALIZATION AS A DEFENCE AGAINST HATRED AND CONTEMPT

It is often said that 'mother' is one of the most beautiful words in the world, and truly it can conjure up within us images of infantile bliss, of warmth, sweetness, peaceful and trustful states such as all of us have known in the past and long for still. This idealized use of the word 'mother' denies the other feelings of terror and hatred that each mother regularly arouses in her child because of her glowering power and her limitless capacity to inflict pain and frustration on her child. It pays tribute to the child's love for the mother and hides the fact that children can and do hate vehemently and frequently. It paints a picture that is too good to be true.

Yet just as the original impetus of our fondness for the serenity of the Madonna-and-child image springs from old infantile experiences and wishes, it is equally true that from the same source springs our fear of witches, with their spells and poisonous magical brews, their evil eyes and their broomsticks, their delight in malice and their greed for children. We know, of course, that both of these infantile derivative images of the mother are absurd and unrealistic and represent accessions of split subjective love and hatred; but I suggest it is something of these two images that interferes with our scientific appraisal of the mothers who come to us for help and leads us massively now to approve, now to disapprove, when we should merely be trying to understand. The child in us, seeking a perfect mother and fearing a bad, is too ready now to idealize, now to blame, and this is an ever-present difficulty in scientific work with mothers.

But this evocative word 'mother' – which highlights the Madonna and shuts out the witch – contains another trick of which we must beware. 'Mother' means simply a woman who has a child, and whose concern is with children. A mother has no man who owns her, or whom she in turn owns and with whom she enjoys a full sexual life to which the child takes second place. In short, a mother is not a sexual *woman*; she is merely a mother. This, too, is the result of the universal childhood wish, to be the one and only interest of the mother, the centre of her world, her only joy, to the exclusion of all and everybody else. The 'father' is also one who has been stripped of sexual joy. He is allowed to have existence only in so far as he is additional property of the child, but he and the mother are not allowed to own each other. The Madonna-mother has no man; nor has the witch-mother; and neither has a sexual life. The mother never has sexual intercourse and it was not passion for and love of a man that made her baby as a by-product. She wanted tenderly to love a baby from the first, and any intercourse that occurred was only to make a baby; the man was a mere accessory, at most, to an act essentially parthenogenetic.

These childhood views, absurd and unrealistic though they be, have inevitably coloured some of our researches up to date. We even talk and think in terms of father, mother, and child rather than of husband, wife, and child; that is to say, we use infant-centred and sexless words rather than adult-centred and sexual ones – a tribute to the ease we all find in being infantile and to the difficulty we find in being adult.

This childish refusal to countenance sexuality in the parents has been found by psycho-analysis to be one of the central human defences against pain. Few of us can imagine our parents wrapped up only in each other, lustily enjoying sexual intercourse – and particularly our mothers. For behind the desperate idealized image of the Madonna lies another fearful creature – the prostitute-mother, who prefers a man to a baby and who is lustful and fiercely happy in sexual congress. Such a picture, which leaves the baby at the mercy of loneliness, rage, murderous jealousy, and helpless dependence on a traitor, small and impotent and unimportant, no longer the centre of the universe but painfully small fry, is intolerable. Various desperate mental defences against this state are quickly erected and one is the denial of the parents' mutual pleasure. The Madonna, sweet, immaculate, gentle – that is our model for a proper mother; and we are her one and only, and she is ours.

In this way, mothering is sterilized and ennobled – or, to put it in another way, it becomes a two-body problem, regressively freed from the danger of having directed towards it the feeling derivatives of the three-body Oedipus situation – envy, anger, contempt, blame, denigration, murder, and jealousy.

To sum up at this stage, our knowledge of mothering is derived much from infant-centred thinking and research, so that our scientific literature on mothering is richly concerned with the problems of the child and but little with those of the wife-mother. This bias derives from two universal human needs: first, to view the childhood self as the centre of the universe, and, second, to retreat regressively from childhood sexual problems to the safety of mother-child thinking.

This regressive emphasis on mothering as of importance to the child, and as a two-body rather than a three-body matter, hinders the view of motherhood as a development in femininity, as a feat of sexual maturity, as an aspect of genitality. Nevertheless, the treatment of women who fail as mothers compellingly shows that mothering capacity marches hand in hand with psychosexual development.

GUILT ABOUT FEMININITY

The taboos of the Oedipus situation laid on the little girl are strengthened by her own persecutory anxiety about her mother whereby she comes to feel that her mother hates her sexual interests as destructively as she hates her mother's. The disappointment of incest wishes and the guilt and anxiety about being in sexual rivalry with her mother lay a blight on the development of frank enjoyment of sexuality and maternality. With growth into womanhood this guilt remains and becomes the invariable companion of wishes for sexual enjoyment. Encouragement and goodwill from others that she should enjoy her husband are much needed by her to counteract this sense of guilt about enjoyments connected with sexuality. If her sense of guilt is massive it will prevent those reassurances from being effective and prevent her from enjoying anything connected with sexual pleasure; indeed, it will produce active aversion to anything remotely connected with it. Evanescent sexual pleasure is one matter, however. Going further and permanently into adult sexuality and actually bearing a child is another. Maternity tests the whole system of the early hidden rivalries and guilts of the Oedipus situation and of the mental defences against these. Maternality, the final sexual achievement of the girl, therefore, carries with it the greatest potential for arousing the hatred of the internalized Oedipal mother-rivalry and for producing a sense of crushing guilt and anxiety. Where the guilt-laden woman was liable to be anxious, or frigid, or hostile to her husband, she will now also be averse to her baby (as a sexual product), and those who encourage her to enjoy one or both will be felt as tempters, asking her to commit destructive sins from which she has turned away in horror.

There are various ways in which human beings deal with guilt, but one common way of surmounting the guilt of sexual enjoyment is to suffer severely and thus placate the rage of the forbidding mother who was internalized in childhood and who remains alive for ever within the mind. This suffering can take any form, but usually it centres on womanhood being burdensome, so that the woman is aloof from feminine enjoyment and unable to co-operate happily with those who seek enjoyment with her. She is unable to enjoy and advance in feminine achievement as a sexual woman and as a mother, to take and give pleasure in her strength of body, her vagina, her breasts and nipples, her milk, her limbs, her warmth, and her adult powers of loving. Enjoyment and activity of those aspects of her body and mind are banned to her, along with pride in herself as a wife who can make her husband sexually happy or as a mother who can produce a lusty and passionate child. Thus, sexual intercourse and later pregnancy have to be matters for shame and suffering, labour for torment and terror, puerperium for weakness, discomfort, and drudgery. As her baby thrives she has to retreat rapidly from any suspicion of pride or pleasure in him and to emphasize the work and trouble he gives her. If anyone praises him she quickly has to show what a nuisance he is, to emphasize the sacrifice and exhausting effort he costs her. Only if she suffers steadily may she be allowed to continue with either her wifely or her maternal life.

In certain women, guilt about genital activity is savagely severe, too great to be atoned for by mere suffering in a setting of marital and maternal stability. Where there is massive guilt the very marriage and the maternity themselves have to be quite wrecked and a much greater degree of suffering must ensue, together with a full renunciation of all pleasures of adulthood, and a return to childlike innocence and obedience. The clinical state of such women is one of helpless suffering and depression, which takes many forms, but in which certain features are constant.

First, the mother, far from enjoying her baby, hates him, puts him from her, is afraid of him, averse to him, or, at least, apathetic about him. She is unable to own him fully and fiercely as her own and she may feel that he is not really hers, in spite of her knowledge to the contrary. She is in no position now to listen to tempting remarks that she should enjoy him, or to defend herself from accusations that she ought to do better with him. She is wide open to criticisms and all too ready to believe that she is ill-equipped for motherhood, that she feeds or attends the baby too little or too much, too rarely or too often. She is all too ready to believe that others would make better mothers than she and are better fitted for the task. Passively she will let strangers look after the baby, and take him from her, or she will seek openly or in more subtle ways for them to do so. If, in their concern for the baby – a matter I shall examine later – her advisers propose that another should look after him, she is very ready to agree. A nurse, a mother, a mother-in-law, an aunt, a sister, a neighbour – any figure who can represent the archaic mother whose rival she has become in the act of giving birth – may now have the baby. After the baby is given to another woman (usually an older one) the patient retreats from rivalry with her.

Second, the mother with severe guilt about having a baby often becomes unable to stand her husband or home. They are now felt as burdensome and distasteful, dirty and demanding. Cooking, cleaning, and other wifely or maternal functions are now not pleasurable but exhausting – to be undertaken with suffering and anxiety. Sexual life with her husband is painful, burdensome, merely to be endured or impossible to undertake. The husband is intolerable, selfish in his wishes for pleasure, and there are quarrels and scenes. Sometimes the husband is told to find another woman, that is, he, too, is renounced to another. The guilt about having the child has thus to be paid for by the sacrifice of others.

Third, the mother retreats from adult life with its forbidden pleasures and its guilt-laden conflicts into a state of anxious, childlike helplessness. Unable to look after home, husband, or child, she seeks instead to be looked after, to be fed, sheltered, and instructed. She is helpless, innocent of ambition or adult responsibility, depressed and unable to take decisions for herself. In extreme states a surrender of the ego occurs with insane retreat to childhood ways in the form of helplessness akin to that of a newborn. Like her own infant, such a mother does not recognize people or things, cannot feed herself, is incontinent, is innocent of time-sense, of simple perception, and has neither co-ordinated purposeful movement nor a securely established body image. Such patients have an anxious appeal for their nurses different from that of all other psychotic patients. Tenderness and gentle concern are faithfully given them without effort or strain, and without any of the fears or impatience induced by other psychoses. They indeed evoke from their nurses the same tender, altruistic attitude as does a newborn child.

Disturbance in the puerperium of this order is well known to medicine and, although it is not common, it is also recognized by the law, which makes special provision for mothers whose rejection of maternity leads them to infanticide. It is as if the law recognizes the right of a woman to flee from success, and to renounce life as a mother. The Mental Treatment Act of 1930 introduced the category of 'temporary insanity', which, although it has been used for other cases, was created especially for those women whose insanity was felt to be a matter for special provision different from all others. Recognition of maternity as a severe test of personality, while general, is not, however, universal. For instance, an outcry in the Press occurs whenever a married woman proposes to give her baby legally to another. The woman is then severely criticized, and tolerant understanding of her plight is not evinced. Indignation, infant-centred, like so much of our research, emphasizes only the baby's needs.

GUILT AND BEHAVIOUR WITH OTHERS

I want now to examine further the fact that a mother is a woman who plainly is wrapped up in a mystery from which we are shut out, a sexual mystery that concerns her own preoccupation with her body at the service of another; this other being, in the first place, the man with whom she lay and whose sperm she took and, now, whose sperm, in the shape of the baby, she still adores, nurtures, and attends.

The fierce intolerance of the child in every one of us for pairing situations, from which we, as children, were shut out, is well known. The envy, anger, jealousy, and denigration, the wish to interfere, to separate the pair, to have each for ourselves, are also well known; it would be surprising therefore if the mother were not surrounded from the first by a host of envious and curious helpers ready to advise and interfere with the sexual act of birth, to be in on the mystery, to prevent her from going about things her own way, to pull the baby out of her vagina, to slap him, to take him from her into another room, to let her have him only sometimes, to ration her enjoyment of him and his enjoyment of her, to advise her how to feed him, wash him, clothe him, hold him, train him, and generally to share her responsibility for him. As I have said, mothers rarely lack helpers and advisers. Simultaneously, the husband, whose very baby it is, may feel something of the same primitive jealousies arising out of the fact that another has taken his beloved and occupies her interest and bodily mysteries in a way that he cannot share. Paternal jealousy of the child is tempered much by the father's identifying with his own child, and if he is secure in his potency he may also much enjoy his role of father (no small feat in itself), but where it is shaky he may regard the baby as his powerful rival. Another kind of jealousy may arise, however. Out of feminine need he may wish to have the baby for himself and resent his wife's possession of the child, so that, as much as any other barren person, he may then sulk, or interfere with the mother's peace of mind by advising her that she is not managing the baby as well as she should, by insisting that he knows best how the infant should be fed. The hatred of the woman's infidelity in taking from, creating, and loving another, makes in general for an ambivalent reception of her maternity.

But the mother herself is, as we have seen, by no means in a position always of personal sureness. She, too, has her need to whitewash the sexual indulgence of intercourse, pregnancy, childbirth, and child-rearing, in order to protect herself from the anger of the mother set up permanently in her unconscious and ready from there to control, spoil, license, and mete out pain and punishment. Once the crime is committed and the long-sought triumph of pregnancy is achieved, the woman needs the sanction of other women and their assurance that she is still loved and not hated and envied. Readily she will seek the company of others like herself and from whom she has little to fear, at maternity clinics and among her pregnant acquaintances, with whom she may make proud jokes about her belly. Elsewhere she may be shy about it as the visible sign of forbidden pleasures, but this depends on how much guilt she carries for rivalry with her own mother in full sexual competition. Some are so secure in adulthood that they need little reassurance about being approved by the sisterhood of women and a few may even openly enjoy the triumph that is theirs over other women, but others may feel that their pregnancy has been stolen behind the back of the world while it was asleep, and may be excessively sensitive to chance remarks of their mothers and mothers-in-law showing envy of their trespass into maternal privilege. Some pregnant women are also very sensitive to the potential envy of their sisters – particularly elder sisters and sisters-in-law, for it is not easily possible for every woman to believe that she has a right to be pregnant and happy.

Women with problems of guilt over this matter are often able to locate in their surroundings a witch-like figure who hates their baby and disapproves of their daring, and they are able indeed to stimulate, by unfriendliness and fear-driven aloofness, certain barren elderly women to adopt this role. It is interesting how often the mother-in-law fills this requirement for them, being regarded as jealous and resentful even though, in fact, she may have much goodwill. It is true, of course, that some mothers-in-law respond readily to the woman's suspicion and prickliness out of their own ordinary envy of maternity and all it means. This envy is the greater because the daughter-in-law is in sexual relation with her own son and has from him a baby that she, because of incest taboos, is prohibited from even daring to wish for. Pregnancy thus places a strain on relations between mother-in-law and daughter-in-law, and if the mother-in-law cannot solve her difficulties by identifying with the young mother, or is shut out by the young mother's fear and hostility, it is true that she may offer pointed advice and sharp disapproval and criticism and be felt as a witch who is jealous of mothers and who wishes to steal their babies and eat them up.

The young mother's fear of the envy and jealousy of other women, especially barren women or those past child-bearing age, is the obverse of her triumph over them and the archaic mother whom they represent. Those women who have internalized early mother images which are approving or tolerant are in little difficulty over this matter – and, indeed, they can turn to their actual mothers, in friendliness and independent love, for tips and reassurance and shared pleasure about the grandchild. But those whose Oedipal relations were stormy and whose internalized mother is savagely crushing of sexuality (in retaliation for her child's savage envy of her own sexuality) cannot be at ease with maternity. They project into the outer world the enraged internal mother whose rights have been usurped and they find her there – in their own mother or mother-in-law. Sometimes, the split mother image of Madonna and witch is distributed between these two maternal figures – from one of which she has, of course, truly taken her husband. One is safe, the other dangerous. At all events, the projection is not difficult to focus on some elderly woman, because some of these are truly ambivalent, like all of us, towards pregnancy and cannot hide all hints of negative feelings towards the young mother in the full flush of her adult sexual privilege.

When persecutory anxiety from enraged maternal images is high, desperate uneasiness and a sense of being in danger drive the young woman towards a slavish need for reassurance that all will be well with her and her baby and that both are still acceptable, lovable, and safe, in spite of her trespass. She is liable now to renounce the triumph of her pregnancy and to feel and emphasize suffering, and thus to appeal for love not as an equal adult but as an inexperienced child who has enjoyed nothing, to be miserable, and to present herself not as one who has pursued sexual deeds but as an innocent victim of a sexual husband who must bear all the guilt. Suffering, sick, and innocent of pleasure, dreading labour in obedience to old guilts, some even renounce their husbands now and go back as obedient erring children who have made a mistake to their mother's house. My colleague, Peter Lomas, who has made a special study of mothering problems and on whose findings I am leaning heavily and freely, has found it common that such young mothers can see their own mothers only as joyless in maternity and drudges of the home. They seem unable to countenance the possibility that their own mothers had any sexual life at all (Lomas, 1959, 1960).

MASCULINE ELEMENTS IN MOTHERING

I now want to turn to another aspect of mothering as a human achievement – that which represents a further step in the overcoming of woman's masculine wishes. You will know that there are several possible determinants of such wishes and that these are of universal application, although they vary in strength with the individual: identification with the father out of a love for him that is felt to have been rejected and frustrated, together with a depreciation of all womanhood including her own; identification with the father out of rivalry with him and of disappointment in not gaining a mother's love; identification with brothers for each of the reasons given above; masculine over-compensation from renunciation of femininity out of fear of internal attacks by a persecuting damaged mother. Such matters lie behind the female rivalry with men that makes for the steady, envious, nagging attacks characteristic of even fairly mature women. In extreme forms they prevent the woman from allowing men and their sexual organs to have any attraction for them and lead to a bitter rivalry instead. In minor forms they prevent the women from marrying a truly masculine man and confine her to a weak one who can be mothered and who will not protect her, but who, at least, prevents her from feeling small and who averts the terror associated with passive surrender to feminine passion.

For women with prominent unsolved problems of this kind, frigidity and domination are the rule. They are unable to love and value men, and pregnancy is felt to be a success in rivalry with men – for it is something singular and important that the envied male certainly cannot himself achieve. It is an opportunity now for the woman to deprecate the man's part in creating the baby, to triumph over him, to show at last that she is as good as or better than he, and has no need of him. She can thus revenge herself for the old bitter disappointments of childhood with men. Usually such a woman overestimates her pregnancy and her children, puts them before all else in her life and drives them on to achieve for herself the distinction that she has felt lacking in all her life. If the child or children are male – so much the better. They will avenge her early hatred of the father, and will beat both him and her brothers – and perhaps her husband as well – in their great achievements, which will owe all to her.

But this way of managing early disappointments in feminine life at the Oedipal period carries a penalty. The little girl who envies and hates the power of men cannot believe that her own masculine achievements can ever be greeted except by a similar envy and hatred from others. Behind the defiant happiness of their masculine triumphs – in this case, pregnancy, birth, the triumphant use of breasts and maternal position – lie uneasiness and a fear of all being attacked by and lost to others. She will abort, she will lose her life in childbirth, her breasts will fail in their function, the baby will prefer his father, she will be once again bereft of masculine power. Such women live in fear of man's envy and resort to the two main systems of behaviour reviewed above – suspicion of the man's ill-will and neglectfulness, accusations about his being not nearly impressed enough with her achievements, complaints about his badness, his unsympathetic lack of support, on the one hand; and, on the other, a declaration that he is lucky and that she is unlucky, that he with his freedom and independence is enviable and that she is not, that he ought to care deeply for her without enmity because she suffers so and has so little joy. If she can ward off the feared envy of men she can permit herself a masculine achievement of giving birth, but her triumph tends to be joyless and bitter – and she may cage herself in arrogance and misery to avert the rage of the internal primitive father whose masculinity she guiltily feels she has stolen. Such women tend to become suffering matriarchs, anxious to have 'good' babies, but limited in their ability to use their femininity. When the child fails to respond to them with enjoyment they become easily depressed, hostile, blaming, or anxious.

Where the baby is a male and thus fulfils the woman's greatest masculine wishes to produce a masculine thing that will make her the equal of any, her relation with the baby is heavily loaded with persecutory fears. The baby's activity, lustiness, and appetite are delightful for her, but this delight is also fearful, for this baby represents the masculine turbulence and violence that she has longed to express all her life and has learned to hide as shameful. With her secret wishes now out, plain in human form for all to see, she needs to control, quell, crush, and banish the very male liveliness before her that others may see and so disapprove of. The pride in her own and her son's masculine vigour is therefore enjoyed only in secret, tortuous ways. Great anxiety, even panic and rage at the baby's wild emotions and demands and at her own failure to keep him quiet and docile, are observable in the severe cases. And complicating all is the envy of the boy and the hostile need to make him like herself, feminine, and unable to enjoy his vigorous maleness. (It is common to hear mothers say, 'Boy babies are far more difficult to manage than are girl babies.' The preoccupation with sexuality that underlies this remark is obvious. I suggest it should be reframed thus: 'It is more difficult *for me* to manage boy babies than girl babies.')

Where problems about masculinity are severe, mental balance may be disturbed. The feminine helplessness and passivity of the birth process may be felt as a loss of command, the attention to the baby at night and the need passively to enjoy and accept the baby's activities and demands as a loss of status. Childbirth may be felt as a loss, and after childbirth a depression may occur. No longer are these women in control of the lump that made them proud and special, and some are afraid that the baby, and not they, will now come first. Maternity is a hideous slavery – everyone fusses over the baby and nobody thinks of the mother. In turn, hatred of the husband for his freedom from such slavery, and of the baby as a rival for importance with others, may ensue. The curse of womanhood and femininity is for these women a painful lot, and the states of depression that follow childbirth, lactation, or weaning may be of psychotic magnitude.

Lastly, you may wonder why I have not concerned myself more with the pregenital anxieties of the puerperium. There are several reasons for this deliberate incompleteness. First, I wanted to examine the common defence against the facts of life, whereby two-body relationships with their subtle but relatively unfrightening pathology are emphasized at the cost of evading the terrifying three-body sexuality of the Oedipus complex. Second, clinical findings in the treatment of disturbed mothers suggest that the appearance of a child is a three-body event of a distinctly sexual order and that disturbances of such apparently pregenital activities as feeding are much less prominent in the clinical picture than is commonly supposed. Third, where pregenital problems do arise, such genital-stage mechanisms as homosexuality and displacement from below upwards should not be ignored. Fourth, I wanted to stress that regression in disturbances of mothering, while certainly related to pre-Oedipal fixation points, occurs because of reactivation of unsolved difficulties in the Oedipus situation, and that they are disturbances of genitality. Thus, while this account is incomplete, at least it re-emphasizes mothering as a development in feminine sexuality, of a three-body order.

16 · *Nursing a Group of Mothers and Children*[1]

BY C. G. M. SCHODT

The group consisted of seven mothers and between them they had ten children. Some of the mothers suffered from depression, some were phobic and could not travel or stay at home by themselves, one had back pains, another urticaria, one felt she would attack children. They all had one additional problem, gross difficulty in caring for their own children.

Most of the families were visited by the psychotherapist or myself before admission. They were admitted to the hospital over a period of two weeks.

A number of other patients were having group therapy at the time, a mixed group of men and women, single girls, and one mother with her child in the hospital. Several other patients with no children were having individual psychotherapy. This paper concerns the interaction of all the patients.

On the first day, the mothers were shown their rooms, met other patients, saw the hospital, and heard something about how it works. They were all accompanied by their husbands. Each mother had a room for herself and her child, except two who had to share. They were to be responsible for their children and had brought cots, washing things, special toys, and any special foods. They knew that we thought they should go home with their children for week-ends.

The group met the doctor for one and a half hours, four times a week, for psychotherapy. The doctor, psychologist, and nurses exchanged information at a weekly meeting, so that the doctor could learn about the patients' lives outside the consulting room

[1] Extracts from a paper published under the title of 'Family-centred Nursing' in the *Nursing Mirror*, 25 November 1960.

and relate this information to what happened in the therapeutic sessions.

The nurse also met the group once a week to discuss practical matters. At times the group members tended to bring up matters more appropriate to the therapeutic sessions and the nurse had to point this out and steer discussion back onto practical lines.

From the first, patients without children resented the mothers, and those with particular difficulties about children complained about the noise and mess. At medical unit meetings, children were usually the topic of discussion, directly or indirectly. The nurse suggested to the mothers that one of them could look after the children during the meetings and that they could work out a rota to do this in turn. But when important matters were known to be coming up for discussion which the mothers apparently did not want to face, they tended to bring their children with them or allowed them to run in and out. Discussion became difficult because of the noise. The nurse would comment when this happened and suggest that the children were being used as scapegoats and as a defence against the unwanted discussion. Then things would improve for a week or so until difficulties would again come up which the mothers wanted to avoid discussing. They would allow the children to run in and out again.

The mothers were sometimes excluded from important jobs in the unit – this was one way for the other patients to show their resentment and for the mothers to isolate themselves. It would be said that they had not been in long enough (even though this was a month after their admission). Not until most of the first group had left did the mothers come into their own and take all the important jobs.

When extra laundering facilities were needed, a bathroom was converted. The mothers liked it but the other patients resented losing what they considered to be one of 'their' bathrooms.

Because the unit was on the second floor, some mothers became anxious that the children might fall over the banisters. The greatest anxiety was expressed by those mothers with strong aggressive impulses towards their children. They seemed to be asking for protection for the children against their feelings. An extra high banister rail was fixed so that any real danger could be reduced. This helped the mothers to recognize that some of the anxiety was within themselves.

A small decorating job was on hand at one time. One of the mothers and her husband decided they would like to redecorate the landing which the patients used as a sitting-room. They chose the colour scheme and bought materials from the unit's allowance. With the help of another patient and her friend and the nurse they decorated the whole landing completely one week-end.

At this time the rest of the hospital was much taken up with a new venture. Patients began to cook their own supper instead of having it done for them by the kitchen staff. Until then, the mothers had been excluded from community work because the other patients felt that they had enough to do looking after the children. But now they were needed. At a general meeting called to discuss this matter, a tremendous amount of resentment between the mothers and non-mothers became clear. The mothers were rejected and felt under attack from everyone. They were allowing too much noise and mess in the dining-room. They stayed too long over meals. They were supposed to have early lunch and leave the dining-room by the time the other patients came in. After stormy discussions, the patients came to an agreement and mothers were included in the rota for making afternoon tea and washing up after supper. They were excused from cooking supper because they would be putting the children to bed at that time.

During their time in hospital, about nine months, feelings between the patients led to various crises. One patient felt she could not stand the group any longer, another did not like the hospital, a third was sure she was better and needed no further treatment. The full resources of the group were needed at these times to help these patients to stay and finish treatment. Later, having found some security and understanding in hospital, most patients felt anxious about leaving. Towards the end of the period, we spent much time discussing problems of discharge. It was decided to undertake a follow-up inquiry three months later. As well as individual improvement, a noticeable change in the mothers was their ability to manage the children differently, with more tolerance and less domination and automatic restriction than they had shown previously.

17 · *The Nursery School*

BY JOAN RUSH

Until April 1962, all the children in the hospital were cared for by their mothers all day, except for an hour's play group provided by the staff. One or two children also attended a nursery school outside. We felt that something more should be provided for children of three to five years of age.

When the school first started, five children attended every day, from 10 a.m. to 3 p.m. They were kept amused and physically cared for, but the day had little structure. It was no more than an extension of the play group and we soon saw that the children needed some routine and direction and, certainly, more play materials.

LEARNING FROM OTHER NURSERY SCHOOLS

My knowledge of how nursery schools were run was limited. I had gained some useful experience in attending the play group run by the psychologist, but I had been working largely with adult patients. I therefore visited nursery schools in the neighbourhood.

I would find a busy, lively group, all seemingly happy and engaged in constructive play, a contrast to our intensely involved small group who spent much time fighting and generally being destructive.

There were differences, too, in how the staff thought about children. On one of my visits, a week before the summer holidays, I asked a teacher how the children felt about the separation. She said that they seldom talked about holidays to the children, that they were just accepted, and that anyway children had no sense of time. This surprised me. I had expected the nursery school staff to be aware of separation problems similar to those of our adult patients and their children. We had spent much time talking with the children about holidays and preparing them for separation. I could see that it might have been inappropriate at times because the child's sense of time is different from that of the adult. Yet it seemed that our children needed to know about, and could be helped to face, separation. They are very much involved with each other all the waking day and their relationships and rivalries are as intense as those between siblings.

Our group was much smaller than those usually found in nursery schools and feelings often ran high. We enlarged the group by including some outpatients' children and 'ordinary' children from the neighbourhood, giving the inpatients' children a wider range of social experience.

Until I visited the local schools we had allowed a lot of free play and permissiveness. But the children needed *known* boundaries. I saw that other schools had very definite boundaries, drawn by trial and error over the years, which worked well. I adopted some of these and found a secure and useful basis to work from. The school day was structured with definite periods for free play, directed activity, lunch, rest, and play in the garden. The children who came after we had structured the day accepted it and adopted its rules as if they had made them themselves. They would say to newcomers whose behaviour was outside the set boundaries, 'We don't do that here!'

This willingness to keep within the boundaries and adopt approved ways of behaviour was, of course, established only after many periods of testing out. At times the whole group would gang up against the teacher. This happened usually when a number of children left at the same time and there would be too few remaining to carry on the culture and initiate the newcomers. Nursery schools generally, not functioning in a hospital setting, can avoid this problem by admitting limited numbers of children at intervals over a period, so that at any one time the majority of the children will have been in the school for many months, but this device is seldom practicable in the hospital situation, where families leave as they become less disturbed and are replaced by families with children often in need of a stable group. The constant nucleus provided by the outpatients' and other children became, therefore, specially important.

The school provides a setting in the hospital where the children can feel free to experience and explore relationships with each other and with the staff, and where mothers can come when needed by the children and can feel they are of some use to them. Children old enough to attend primary school sometimes come to the nursery school. In some cases the child is not yet able to cope with the experience of a large group. Sometimes he clings to the mother or develops school phobia which must be treated before he can go to school. Often it is the mother who has great difficulty in separating from her child and both need help before the child feels free to leave her. Even in cases where the child is less disturbed, it is usually the mother who is the more anxious when the child first attends. Only when she begins to feel more secure can the child begin to feel free to enjoy the school.

A TYPICAL DAY

It is Monday morning, ten o'clock. My assistant and I are ready.

John, aged five, and Susan, his sister, aged four, burst in, without their mother. They usually come on their own except when their mother wants to issue some order to me through them: 'Don't dare get wet today', or 'Keep your sweater clean, John, I'm fed up with washing.' John is in a fighting mood, starts jumping up and down on a rest-bed. I know from a nursing report that his family had a rough week-end at home with much anxiety about leaving, so I am prepared for some trouble.

Richard, aged four, and Michael, his brother, aged six, come in with their mother. Michael immediately gets the pencils out and starts sharpening them (he attends the school during his own school holidays). Their mother leaves suddenly, saying she has to go to a meeting. Richard makes a few tentative stabs towards the toys on the shelf, preparatory, I feel, to sweeping them all on the floor.

I sense that the children need some activity they can all get involved in, and I suggest cooking, which they all enjoy. They get ready, putting on aprons, getting out the rolling-pins.

Pamela, aged two and a half, arrives with her mother, who apologizes for being late. Pamela decides she wants to leave, goes out with her mother, and returns happily about two minutes later. She becomes occupied with cooking.

Everyone is playing with the dough, rolling and making shapes.

John and Richard fight over a rolling-pin but another is found and all is well.

Susan is surreptitiously eating her dough. When everyone has finally moulded his dough and made shapes according to his liking, she has none – she's eaten it all. We find another bit for her and put her initial on it. All the children mark their dough and we all troop out to the kitchen to put it in the oven. John stays there with me to help to get morning drinks. He likes turning the taps on and off for me and makes great efforts to do it well. The others go back to the school and help my assistant to clear up and wash the dishes. John and I return with the drinks.

As we sit and have coffee and lemonade, I ask the children about the week-end. Sometimes they tell me about it, sometimes they say nothing. Today they do not want to talk, they all went nowhere and nothing happened. Susan takes my spoon and keeps it all day in her hand.

After drinks we go into the garden. The children take it in turns to unlock the garden door. Today it is Susan's turn. John is furious, tries to hit her and grabs the key. When I restrain him he runs about the room, very angry, flings himself on a rest-bed, crying loudly, then runs out of the room.

The others go into the garden, taking buckets and spades, and go off to the sandpit. I ring the ward to tell John's mother that he is upset and on his way down to see her. She sounds cross but says she will bring him back. I follow the others into the garden. My assistant is pushing Pamela on the swing. Michael and Richard are digging and Susan is feeding sand to her doll with my spoon.

John appears, dancing and smiling. His mother comes over, fairly well contained, talks to Susan in rather a threatening manner, relents, and is quite warm with Susan and John. She leaves.

Play continues. At one point, Pamela tries to take Susan's (my) spoon and a fierce battle ensues. Another spoon is found. Pamela is not satisfied, flings it down, then says 'Pam's cold' and hugs herself and goes indoors.

At midday we all go in. Michael leaves at this time to return at two o'clock. There is a hustle of going to the lavatory, washing hands, getting out table cloths, arranging tables. Pamela is getting miserable, wants mummy. Her mother arrives, picks her up and cuddles her, and both leave looking pleased with themselves. John rings up Frank, the kitchen porter, on the toy telephone and tells him to hurry up, they are hungry. Frank arrives amid great excitement. 'What is it today, Frank? Is it chips?' They all scramble around me to examine the meal, then sit down impatiently. John teases Susan, says he will eat her dinner. Susan cries and pokes my spoon in his eye. They settle down to eat and all is quiet. My assistant goes to lunch and the children say good-bye to her.

After lunch the children help me to tidy up. John carries out the lunch tins, Susan helps me to fold the cloths and Richard pulls the curtains to. He and John help to get out the rest-beds. Susan jumps on to Richard's bed and he kicks her. She refuses to move until I intervene. Finally they are all on their own beds and I tuck them in, give them their apples and tell them a story. It is usually the same story, with variations that I make up each day. They are all in it and take turns saying their parts. If I leave out a bit they will correct me. Sometimes they quarrel about their parts but usually they enjoy it very much.

They go on munching their apples, looking at books, talking quietly. Sometimes they are sleepy, sometimes noisy and provocative. I go to lunch at this time and hear varying reports when I return.

'Rest' ends and they put their beds away, folding the blankets, putting on shoes. Just before two o'clock, John's mother comes in shouting, 'Come on, John, time to see the lady!' John runs out and bangs the door. Michael returns and gets out the Plasticine. Richard tries to take all of it, but Michael is firm and gives him one bit. Michael makes lots of animals, he models very well. He laughs at my efforts and Richard throws my model on the floor. He starts throwing all the Plasticine on the floor, grabs Susan's doll and throws it in the sink. I ask him to pick up the Plasticine; he refuses; I say it must be done before we go back into the garden. He says he'll do it if I don't look. He often says this, as if he will lose face if I see him obeying my wishes. He picks it all up and we go into the garden.

They all ask for 'a walk in the woods', which they call going around the trees in the garden. I suggest we wait till John comes back; they agree, and sweep the steps until then. John comes back and we all go out, John rushing ahead, jumping on the brambles 'clearing a path'. Michael is interested in birds and trees and can identify all of them. Richard picks up a small branch and starts hitting Susan. I hold his hand and he stops. Then they collect twigs and branches and run back into the school, finding dishes and filling them with water. Susan spills some on her dress and is anxious, starts crying and I reassure her.

Michael gets very excited as he always does just before school ends at three o'clock, runs about the room making noises like a dog.

The mothers come in, I immediately talk to Susan's mother about her dress, feeling I have to protect her. Today her mother is able to smile, is pleased with Susan's offering of twigs from the garden. Michael is prancing around his mother making a lot of noise. Richard is telling his mother that he was the best boy at 'rest' time. They start trailing out when suddenly Michael remembers the cooking. It had been saved from disaster earlier and he brings it out triumphantly. The mothers look dubious but say it looks lovely and they will eat it later. The children go off, shouting, 'Good-bye, see you tomorrow.'

PAINTING, MAKING THINGS, AND DRESSING UP

On other days, the children will decide on some other form of creative play. One day Susan painted a picture of 'a hungry, angry lion who is a bit naughty'. When she started painting she was obviously angry but on being able to put her feelings into the picture she became more relaxed and, in addition, pleased with the praise her picture received.

Cutting out and pasting are much enjoyed by the children. Sometimes the whole group is able to work together and produce a big picture or a scrapbook. At other times the children will work individually. Again, they are provided with an outlet for aggressive feelings while producing a pleasing result.

Dressing up and acting also have great value. They play 'mothers and fathers', or 'hospital', often enacting what has happened. One child will take the role of parent and the dolls or smaller children become 'the children'. Children who have been physically ill, possibly in a hospital, will play doctor or nurse and give injections to the dolls. This way of expressing feelings helps, indirectly, to relieve stress and also offers the nursery school staff some insight into a child's anxiety and preoccupation. It is important that the children be allowed to play these games without stimulation or interference. The staff only rarely need to intervene when a child becomes over-anxious or disturbs the other children. The over-punitive 'mother' or aggressive 'doctor' soon finds that the other children refuse to play the roles allotted to them.

THE HOSPITAL COMMUNITY'S USE OF THE SCHOOL

The school is seen and used by the other sections of the hospital community in many different ways. The mothers themselves may want to be relieved of responsibility and may hope to use the school as a dumping ground. They will push their children through the door in the morning and be late calling for them at the end of the day. Others hope that the children will be disciplined by a strict staff. Some want the children to have some formal teaching, to learn to read and write.

The nurses involved with the mothers are reassured to know that the children of aggressive or neglectful mothers are being cared for. When the mother is particularly ill and finds it hard to care for her child, she may try to exert pressure on the staff to admit a child below the usual age limit. Sometimes we are asked to allow children recovering from the usual childhood ailments to return early so that the mothers can give more time to younger siblings.

Demands come from the children, too. One child literally referred herself for admission, a precocious two-year-old, nearing the admission age, whose mother wanted to keep her as a baby. She would come down the garden and press her nose to the window, demanding to be let in. With encouragement from the nursing staff, her mother eventually agreed that she could attend in the mornings.

There is always an unspoken demand from the hospital as a whole to keep the children entertained, quiet, and out of the way. When they shout and tear about the hospital, the school staff will be told, '*Your* children are making a lot of noise today!'

COMMUNICATION CHANNELS

The school developed alongside other changes in the hospital and a need for new channels of communication was demonstrated. At first the school staff had two channels of communication with the rest of the hospital, one with the nursing staff and one with the mothers. Communication with the nurses was irregular and was usually confined to exchanging information about new admissions. The formal time set aside for communication was the weekly nursing meeting with the matron, where general problems took up much of the time. The children's problems would be contained in the school while the family problems were retained by the staff involved with the mothers, and the two were kept separate. I attended the weekly mothers' meeting, however, and could use some of this time to talk with the mothers about their children.

The school continued to operate in this relative isolation until the following year, when communication was extended by the institution of a weekly meeting between the school staff and all the nursing staff who were involved with the mothers and children. The mothers' meeting was replaced by another meeting for mothers whose children were attending the school. Occasional evening meetings were also held so that the fathers could be involved.

By September 1964 meetings between the school staff, psychotherapists, and other nurses were taking place as a matter of routine. The observations and reports of the school staff were now used in the assessment of families and their progress in the hospital.

We learned much about the needs of parents, children, and staff when the nursery school was established.

First, we learned the need for an organizational structure in which the roles and relationships of parents, children, and staff could be defined. The stable group of parents and children helped to continue the culture established, but changes and adaptations will be needed according to the needs of new participants. Second, boundaries of permitted behaviour for the children and the adults (patients and staff) had to be defined.

Third, and perhaps most important, procedures for dealing with situations were evolved through meetings and through the daily work of those concerned. For example, the co-operation of a mother in recognizing the importance of parting from and reunion with her child was more easily obtained once we had an established procedure. The child is told clearly what days and what times he will be in school and when his mother will fetch him. This is repeated with the school staff so that the child knows that the adults are agreed. The child's trust in adults is the more supported if the mother can be helped to co-operate by bringing and taking the child at the agreed times. The school staff can prepare the child for the end of the day and reunion with the mother, family, and hospital community by talking about what they may all be going to do when the mother comes. In this way, the child's emotional investment in people can be transferred from school to family relationships.

18 · Nursing Disturbed Adolescents

BY DOREEN MARTIN

For many years adolescents were occasionally admitted to the hospital, usually one or two at a time, more rarely as a group. The ensuing chaos involving staff, patients, and the neighbourhood made us despair of trying to treat them. After further reflective study of the problems in detail, however, we felt they had taught us enough about the pitfalls for us to begin again.

By 1963 we felt ready to open an adolescent unit. The nurses shared their apprehension about dealing with young people in discussion with other staff. Persistent opposition came from many quarters, but plans went ahead, with some increasing confidence.

Eight boys and eight girls, none under fifteen years, were admitted over a period. Our chief problem, asserting itself in all kinds of situations, became that of integrating the youngsters in the total hospital community and guarding against the unit's isolation.

Three rules, specific to the adolescents, were felt by the staff to be necessary for the 'caring framework' against which they might rebel without too much danger. We knew we should have battles but felt we could, at least, choose the battleground. The adolescents were:

(1) to be in hospital by 10.30 at night
(2) to be in their bedrooms by midnight
(3) to drink no alcohol.

Gradually the rules took on a life of their own, being owned neither by the nurses, the doctors, nor the adolescents themselves. They became meaningless, broken regularly, with the nurse feeling incompetent, frustrated, angry, and ready to blame the doctor for not taking action, and the doctor feeling and saying that it was a nursing problem.

COMMUNITY INVOLVEMENT

The problem only began to solve itself when we put it to the community: How do we contain sixteen adolescents in this hospital? The adult patients were furious at what they felt to be staff incompetence. But they increased their executive committee to include two adolescents.

The constitution, drawn up by the patients and modified over the years as the community develops, now contained a new clause:

> 'If a patient is unable to participate in the community this is destructive both to himself and to the community and he will be unable to benefit from community therapy. The following expectation has therefore been made: it is reasonable to expect adolescents to be in the hospital by 11 p.m., and other members by midnight.'

This is the only specific difference between what is expected of adolescents and what is expected of adults. But instead of anti-social behaviour being tackled only by the staff, the whole community now sees and feels its effects and is involved in dealing with it.

Sandra, for example, aged seventeen, had obsessional traits. She refused to attend meetings and stopped doing her share of domestic work, using her fear of 'contamination' as her reason. The community was patient and made allowances. Special meetings would be arranged for her. In time, patience ran out and the community offered her two weeks to make up her mind whether she stayed and took part in community life or left. For ten days, there was no obvious response. The next evening, Sandra was cold-shouldered at a party and saw this as the end of the road. The following morning she came to the meeting and offered some constructive advice to a fellow patient. She was allowed a new beginning.

We expect adolescents to continue their schooling or find part-time work, and many of our nursing problems lie in dealing with their reluctance to attend school or get to work. An added difficulty is that of finding part-time work locally. Inability to work is often a pointer to the patient's disturbance and we place emphasis on the carrying out of tasks in the hospital work groups.[1] Comment will be made by patients who are inconvenienced by the lack of work of one of the members of their group. The value of such comment lies not in its criticism of an individual but in that it allows the injured

[1] See also Chapter 20 – Ed.

and injuring parties to understand the effect they have on each other, particularly important for the adolescent who is working out his problems of social responsibility.

We try to modify gang behaviour constructively. In the work groups every patient has the chance to become manager, a post offering opportunity to learn about responsibility and having real authority. The patients' constitution puts it thus:

> 'He is responsible for calling meetings, initiating and controlling discussion, allocating work and ensuring it is done, being generally responsible for the group and reporting any particular difficulties of individuals back to the morning meeting.'

The week-end problem, unlike that of other institutions caring for adolescents, is not of absconding but of leaving the hospital to go home. Working through separation anxieties, in relation to the hospital or the home, occupies much of our attention.

Other problems centre on 'rooming', as we call it. The patients' housing committee allocates rooms and this opens up opportunities for examining the very real difficulties of sharing.

When Desmond, aged seventeen, applied to change his room, he complained to the committee that his room-mates were teasing him and making him do all the cleaning. His room-mates for their part claimed that he asked for it because of his provocative talk and behaviour. They all agreed to try sharing for another two weeks, the chairman recommending that tolerance on both sides might be useful. At the end of two weeks, however, two adult patients offered an empty bed in their room to Desmond. The housing committee, first satisfying itself that everyone had made an effort, agreed to the change, with another recommendation that Desmond and his ex-room-mates attempt to understand the episode in their therapeutic sessions.

The adolescents' spontaneity, warmth, sudden enthusiasms, and outspokenness offer nursing rewards as enjoyable as they are fleeting. The special contact they have with younger children is a good example. One Christmas, as a surprise, they spent hours rehearsing the young children for a nativity play, making their own costumes and scenery. The play was a delight to watch. It lasted only five minutes but the youngsters loved having this secret from the grown-ups and giving them, the mothers especially, such obvious pleasure.

INVOLVING THE PARENTS

Anyone working with adolescents also knows the guilt and anxiety they arouse. We try to use these feelings as a guide to the understanding of what is going on inside the youngster and of the kind of response he evokes in his parents. How can the home situation change along with the adolescent who is receiving treatment designed to help him to change, unless the parents have a chance to understand some of these feelings themselves? By admitting an adolescent to hospital, we may be playing to the parents' feelings of worthlessness, inadequacy, and guilt. The hospital will be seen by them as the 'better' parent. We may collude in this ourselves. To help to deal with such problems we began parents' groups.

Our basic approach relies on the well-tried formula of attempting to see the disturbance of the presenting patient within the whole family pattern. During the outpatient assessment, the doctor will see parents and child together, then interview the child alone, before deciding whether to recommend admission, and the nurse will visit the home requesting that all the family be present.

Some adolescents have no home. They have rejected, or been rejected by, their parents. Some are orphans and may come to us from welfare institutions. We try, then, to see and keep in contact with an adult (aunt, foster parent, grandmother, welfare officer) who has a fairly stable relationship with the patient and is trusted by him. For example, 'my guardian', as one of the adolescents calls the children's officer, attends the weekly parents' group. Another's probation officer visits regularly. Some patients refuse any offers of contact with anyone older, parent or not. Some parents consistently refuse contact with their child or the hospital. Such situations present particularly difficult nursing problems during the inpatient period and after discharge. But they tell us much about the family disturbance.

It is hospital practice never to discuss a patient with his relatives unless he is present and has given his consent. The parents' group takes its structure from this practice. In its present form it will consist of eight adolescents, boys and girls, their parents or an adult *in loco parentis*, and a nurse. The nurse has a multiple role in the group. She convenes it, represents the hospital and its staff, facilitates the work of the group, intervening when appropriate. She will often see disturbance in the parents. She does not try to tackle this herself but will give the information to the doctor, perhaps for referral to the outpatients' psychiatric social worker.

The group encourages parents to involve themselves in their children's treatment. They gain some relief through discussing their problems in a supporting situation where their worries will be echoed by other parents, perhaps even by their own child. They share the difficulties created by their child and can begin to understand his problem of being an inpatient. Discussion often centres on how far the parents feel they can trust the hospital or understand its methods. One parent has heard rumours that his son is stealing, another believes overt sexual relationships are permitted, another discovers her daughter has a bill to pay for smashing a window. At such times they want to know: 'What are *they* (the hospital authorities) doing about it? Why don't *they* put a stop to it?' Here the nurse will attempt to show how unreal is such a demand; she will try to help the parents to see that they and the hospital are involved together and share the same anxieties. When both 'good' and 'bad' parents are brought together it is immaterial who is playing which role at the time, and we are able to explore situations together as they arise with all the people involved. Real and current problems will be discussed: week-ends, work and earnings versus pocket money, holidays, school work and examinations, adolescent sexuality and aggression.

NURSING PROBLEMS

Many people working with adolescents seem to get vicarious satisfaction from it and are tempted to dwell at length and in vivid detail on the problems they present. There is a temptation for such workers to isolate themselves from other workers and develop a closed in-group of people 'with special understanding and sensitivity'.[1] They form an in-group not unlike the adolescents' own gang. It seems to be yet another reflection of what is going on inside the adolescent in his search for an identity.

Discovery of a split between the parents, or between them and the hospital, puts the staff on guard for a similar split among themselves, with the patient perhaps widening it and certainly becoming confused and distressed himself. Observations, information, ideas, agreements, and, above all, disagreements, have to be shared and

[1] See Chapter 5 – Ed.

understood in the staff group looking after adolescents. The group, in turn, must be in regular communication on such matters with the other staff, with the patients' families, with outside agencies such as general practitioners, probation officers, and children's officers, if it is not to become a split-off, self-justifying 'gang'.

The rapidly developing emotions and attitudes of adolescents make great demands on the nurse. Recognizing her involvement with the adolescents makes the enlarging of her skills the more important. She becomes a 'barometer' at times, registering feelings, then moving back to interpret them in terms of the emotional development of children. In a group, the nurse will offer for discussion, for example, her discovery of two youngsters petting in a bedroom. She at once finds herself under attack. 'What a dirty-minded old woman! We weren't doing anything. You *never* understand us!' Surprised at the sudden, intense hostility and at her own angry response, she is uncertain what to do, despairs of work continuing at the moment, but tries to use her own feelings to understand the situation. Perhaps her own anger reflects that of the child, still in the adolescent and in herself, angry when his gratification is interrupted; her own uncertainty, that of the child uncertain about using appropriate times and places for his performances; her own despair, that of the child feeling his mother's criticism as a withdrawal of love. She can then help the group's work to go on. She may ask why the two youngsters demonstrate their feeling for each other in the hospital when they know such behaviour is open to discussion. Put back to the group, the topic can be considered at an adult level in terms of people's responsibilities for each other.

The nurse herself gains support in the learning situation provided by the routine discussion with nursing colleagues. She will hear how others would have dealt with a similar situation, and is free to criticize, comment, or question, so clarifying her own technique.

The years of adolescence, intensely exciting, fearful, awkward, charming, happy, miserable, are a search for identity, separate from that of the external parents, while establishing parental figures securely within, so that a new place may be found in the family.

Some idea of this can be illustrated by what happened to James, an intelligent boy, studying for A-level examinations and working on Saturdays for pocket money. He belongs to a large family, and his parents find it difficult to manage with increasing economic and social demands. James took over a managing role in the family, settling his sisters' quarrels about food, helping his mother with 'best buys' in the market. When his father began to lose time at work because of headaches, however, James felt hopeless and lost, and attempted suicide. After a period in another hospital, James found the community life of the Cassel a great challenge. He was soon elected chairman of the works committee, and later of entertainments. He took charge of buying food for the patients. When the record player needed mending and there was no money, he organized a successful collection.

In effect, he took the role he had made for himself at home, a kind of combined parent figure, on the pattern of the childhood phantasy that the parents cannot manage on their own and the child has to organize them. This 'stealing' of a role means that the internal parents are undermined and made helpless, while the child triumphantly thinks he can 'do it better'. An internal instability of this nature inevitably leads to the danger of the kind of collapse that James had already experienced. This time, patients and staff could try to show him what he was doing, and that the hospital would not collapse if he gave up his role of organizer-in-chief; others could take it on just as well.

James found it very hard to be deprived of his so-called responsibility and to face his depression. This is the kind of situation where the parents' group is a great help. The adolescent can begin to see how other people have struggles, conflicts, frustrations, and a sense of failure, not so different from his own. In the discussions of a problem such as the one described, parents and children can begin to understand something about taking responsibility, that this is not the prerogative of either sex or age, but is different at various stages of development.

Mark Twain wrote, 'When I was a boy of fourteen, my father was so ignorant, that I could hardly stand to have him around. When I was twenty-one, I was astonished how much he had learned in seven years.' James's experience was not unlike this.

19 · *Nursing Families*[1]

BY JANICE WEBSTER

The hospital community, having grown accustomed to mothers with small babies and toddlers, and to husbands and older children as frequent visitors, found that including complete families in the day-to-day life caused its own strains.

After a day at work, the husbands wanted relaxation in the evenings, as well as an investment in community affairs. A spontaneous baby-sitting service, initiated by the married couples and later incorporating the single patients, came to be used as a practical way of repayment by the younger people to the couples for 'parental' support. Husbands also became active in demanding more realistic provision of comforts by the patients for each other. For example, they complained, loudly and without hesitation, if patients preparing the evening meal were slovenly in their job. At the same time, the husbands stimulated other patients, both directly and by example, to increase contacts with society outside. With baby-sitting shared, the couples could make more use of local amenities and would often take some younger patients along. The husbands, too, often offered useful suggestions and support to single patients seeking part-time jobs while in hospital.

The school-age children admitted with their parents did not create any immediate problems. Laundering and cooking facilities had already been provided for the mothers. But seven- and eight-year-olds do not stay as close to mother's skirts as do toddlers. The community had to adapt to the explorations, demands, naughtiness, and curiosity of the school-age child; to deal with the rivalry the child part of each adult experiences when in close contact with

[1] Adapted from a paper published under the title of 'Nursing Families in a Therapeutic Community' in the *International Journal of Nursing Studies*, Vol. 3, pp. 1–7, 1966.

many children; to formulate a broad policy around the sanctions allowed by parents for the immediate, sensible discipline of these older children by the community 'aunts and uncles'. To allow parents time for meetings and discussion groups, the community joined in planning and stocking play areas for the children and shared responsibility for supervision of play groups.

Contact with the local community was increased by the statutorily required links with local junior and secondary schools. Mothers out shopping would meet local mothers to whom they had often been introduced by their children at the school gates. The children from the hospital and the neighbourhood invited each other to tea.

Families in the hospital gave the nurse new opportunities to observe the family as a biological and socio-psychological unit, to know and understand a little about the individuals, how they relate to and use each other in the family, and how the family, as a system containing separate people, relates to the hospital community and the nurse herself.

Families, each being unique, are difficult to categorize, even roughly; but two types of mother have been described by Doreen Weddell: first, women who were ill before marriage and whose illness now disturbs the whole family, and, second, women who have become ill as a result of a specific event – e.g. childbirth. She also identified another type of family problem which presents an acute relationship difficulty, usually between one pair of its members.[1] Quite often, the difficulty in this paired relationship has brought the whole family to the point of fragmentation or, at times, to the threatened or actual exclusion of one disturbed and disturbing member. A husband may be on the point of leaving home, or a child of being sent to a boarding-school or special school for disturbed children.

The nurse's routine first contact with a family in its own home offers opportunity to clarify many of the practical difficulties of the projected move to hospital and begins the nurse-family group relationship. The way in which the nurse is received in her role as visitor-observer allows her some impression of the family's social adjustment and a first assessment of some of the pressures and interrelationships around the presenting 'sick' member. Many family members have some awareness of their involvement in the

[1] See Chapter 14 – Ed.

presenting patient's symptoms, but, in some cases, one of the nursing tasks at the home visit is to recognize and attempt to deal with their resistance to becoming involved in treatment.

For example, a mother and child had been referred from a child guidance clinic because of their engagement in an invidious perpetual war over toilet-training. The little girl stubbornly soiled her own and her siblings' clothes and the mother had attacked the child so furiously that the neighbours had twice called in the NSPCC.[1] The two boys were at home with their parents, the two girls (the elder of whom was the referred child) had been farmed out with neighbours. At the outpatient medical consultation the whole family was offered admission – both the parents and all the children – but the father refused the offer of accommodation and treatment for himself. At the home visit, the nurse learned that both parents had family histories of broken homes and deprived childhoods in which they had been physically maltreated. The nurse realized that the family had fragmented to the point where the father was 'wholly good' and the mother 'wholly bad', and that both colluded in this picture of themselves. The mother was presented with a *fait accompli.* The father had allowed the lease of the house to lapse and had arranged lodgings for himself. He seemed to presume that the hospital would take over his family problems and return the family with the problems magically solved some time later. The nursing at once became centred on an attempt to help the father to own his involvement with his family's difficulties and to value his potential contribution to its treatment.

On admission, each family's method of functioning determines the manner and pace of its integration in the hospital community. In addition, of course, current community pressures and preoccupations contribute to the ease or difficulty of the new people's acceptance. The nurse helps the acceptance as best she can by family and community discussion. She will be with the family and will discuss difficulties as they arise, but she will not give direct advice or take over the problem. She sees her task as enabling the mobilization of the community's nursing potential. A mother with feeding difficulties, for instance, will be supported by other mothers who have culturally sanctioned power and means to organize a rota so that someone can be with the mother at difficult times. The husband, too, will find cultural support from the community to

[1] National Society for the Prevention of Cruelty to Children.

continue his role of breadwinner and to retain the responsibility and authority inherent in his position in the family.

Husbands and wives have themselves created a formal discussion group meeting once a week, to which a nurse is invited. A conglomerate of subjects is discussed, opinions are offered, compared, and contrasted, and actions planned. One couple had problems of discipline with their children. The mother had withdrawn all vestige of authority, the father taking over both parental roles in this respect. They were able, through discussion, to see their parental authority as having value for their children and could begin to share this responsibility with each other in practice. After some time, they even became helpful to some of the adolescent patients in difficulties over the hospital ruling that they must be in the building by 10.30 in the evening.

Children are a joy and a nuisance to all adults, including nurses. Throughout a family's stay in hospital, the children remain wholly the parents' responsibility. This demands special self-discipline and skill on the part of the nurse. She must learn to recognize and understand the wish of the mother to regress and be cared for herself, and yet not be tempted automatically to take over the children – no matter how appealing – when the mother declares she cannot cope. On the other hand, the nurse must not deny that at critical points the mother may need temporary relief, perhaps for an hour or two a day. The nurse's task, however, is not to take over but to encourage the give and take of support between the mothers themselves. Discussion between the mothers about their children can often help a mother to accept the special difference between her own children and others, irrespective of whether or not this is felt to be due to her and her husband's handling. The actual observation of other parents' similar difficulties, and of their varied methods of managing them, frequently opens the way for a mother to examine her own techniques, maybe to improve on them, without resort to the nurse as the 'expert', which carries with it the implication of the mother's failure.

A particular requirement for the nurse, therefore, is to be aware of pressure to collude with the parents' wish to regress and hand over their problems. By her understanding of the child's need for his family, she will appreciate the possible deleterious effects on the child and the family if she replaces the parental authority with her own. This understanding helps the nurse to work with the healthy part of the parents' functioning, to respect their position in the family, and to underline this by taking care always to relate to and address them with the equality due to them as responsible adults. The traditional nursing satisfaction of being, in phantasy, the 'good mother' is replaced by the more adult, subtle satisfaction of supporting a family to retain its adult integrity. A similar temptation for the nurse may arise if the married couple, or one member of it, tries to form a special, separate relationship with her. Here again, the nurse's task, and satisfaction, is to aid the couple to retain responsibility for their problems between themselves, the nurse and other couples being accessible for discussion if they want it.

The cultural norm for families to return home for week-ends presents practical difficulties for those with many children, but it is generally welcomed and seems valuable in retaining the links with the environment from which the family came and to which it will return. The children keep in touch with home surroundings and friends and the parents can test out the shared experience of hospital life against the background to which they will be discharged. The family is not desocialized by a continuous stay in hospital but care must be taken over their resocialization. Hospital practice is for the family and staff to decide jointly the date of discharge some weeks beforehand, so that throughout the remainder of their stay the parents will have the community's support in arranging the practical details and opportunity to discuss and share some of the fears and anxieties about returning home. The social worker and health visitor from the family's district visit the hospital frequently before the discharge date for linking discussions with the family and the hospital nurse.

During a family's hospitalization, the psychiatrist, the nurses, the child therapist, and the nursery school staff work as a team, meeting often, keeping in close touch with each other's points of view, work anxieties, and problems in respect of each family. The individual team member's reactions to the family will be used to increase understanding of the family. Particular care is taken to bring out any disagreement within the team about the family, for staff disagreements often reflect similar disagreements in the family itself. The sharing of stress by the team can subsequently allow a sharing of the satisfactions when a family can remain intact through a critical period of its development, with its equilibrium restored and, optimally, its level of functioning improved.

20 · *Community Nursing*

BY HAZEL EDWARDS

Interest in community nursing led to many developments in nursing practice. One of the most important was that of discussing nursing problems with the patients instead of only among the nursing staff. It was not easy for anyone but it helped the patient to maintain responsibility for himself and other patients, and, to some extent, mitigated the feelings of the nurse that her job was to manipulate the environment for the greater comfort of herself and the patient. It helped both nurse and patient to see that, through understanding something of each other's difficulties, and in working together on the problems each created for the other, they were sharing a task which could bring mutual satisfaction. Each could learn something from the other about a current situation and the occasion for it, and had an opportunity to work out a new solution.

For example, Sarah, a patient with severe eating difficulties, was nursed in the community. With her permission, the nursing problem was presented to the community meeting. She could not eat normally. She collected food scraps in her locker, cooked messes at night, gobbled them up, and vomited afterwards. She lied about food and was losing weight.

The mothers immediately responded and offered to supervise her meals and help her. For a time all went well and the mothers could report progress. Then Sarah began 'misbehaving again', as the mothers put it. She was nibbling bits of food stowed away in secret. She screamed abuse and dissolved into tears if anyone tried to stop her. She took advantage of kitchen duty to raid the waste bins. When the patients relieved her of kitchen duty she got herself elected to the catering committee so that she had legitimate reason for visiting the food store and kitchens.

The patients were exasperated with and sorry for her in turn and, inevitably, there was some punitive response. The ambivalence to the nursing role was shown when it was learned that some patients were secretly giving food to Sarah. It was more subtly expressed when they elected her to the catering committee before she could personally control her eating habits.

In the community meeting, the frustration and anger of Sarah, other patients, and the staff could be shared and, to some extent understood. Sarah was antagonizing the very people she needed to maintain responsible roles with her. The mothers were anxious but did not want her to get into trouble with the staff. They felt that their good mothering was threatened. Like the special nurse with the special patient,[1] they responded by giving more time, more attention, only to be faced with failure, leading to their guilty withdrawal. But the community held firm. The fact that Sarah, even in the stormiest phases, was able to appreciate that people were trying to help and understand, made the situation tolerable. Her gradual improvement was a relief and satisfaction to everyone. The community could provide a reasonably stable environment which could contain the acting out without dividing itself into hostile camps supporting one view or another.

Four times a day patients and staff meet to share problems and find ways of living and working together – in the morning, in the afternoon, and in early and late evening. The meeting at 6.30 p.m. is attended by husbands and the younger people back from work, the children back from school, and the evening duty nurse. At this meeting, areas of tension can be identified and the events of the day reviewed, so that distress can be supported before it develops into violent acting out.

The last meeting is at ten o'clock when the evening nurse and the patients' representative meet to review the evening and prepare their report for the morning. This evening procedure developed from the patients' criticism of the way in which the nurses presented their reports. The nurses, too, were dissatisfied with this. The patients decided to elect a representative to be 'on duty' with the nurse every evening. Both could then report back jointly to the community meeting.

This arrangement of meetings provides a continuity in the life of the community and, in a practical sense, has helped to centre the nurses' interest on the community and the groups within it.

[1] See Chapter 5 – Ed.

WORK GROUPS

The community, accepting a recommendation from the patients' executive committee, decided that everyone should be included in a work group. Each group would have about fifteen members, comprising one or two complete families, three or four single adults, five or six adolescents, and two nurses, a senior and a junior. Each group, with an elected works manager, is responsible for maintaining, cleaning, and decorating a particular area of the hospital, and for arranging its own work programme. Actual work or devising a work programme may be delayed if a group is preoccupied with some other matter, as the following examples show.

One day, a group continued discussing a problem already explored in the community meeting, that of a mother unable to look after her child. Some searching for someone to blame led to the question, 'Why don't the nurses do something?' At this point, the nurse could have pursued the problem of the apparently neglectful mother and explored with the group the resources in the community available to mothers needing help. But her task in this situation was to help the group to get on with its own task of planning the work for the morning. She asked what arrangements the group was going to make. The group felt that it could not get on because some members had not turned up. It was divided in opinion about one absent member: 'He can't help staying away, he's sick' versus 'We're sick too but we come to work just the same'. Again, the nurse could have indulged in an interesting chat about the meaning of absenteeism or she could steer the group towards the less fascinating topic of getting the rooms cleaned. She said, 'Well, what about *our* problem?' The works manager then took command, asked for volunteers to bring the absentees to the meeting, and began allocating jobs. The nurse's task was now to help the group to own the work requirements and to support the works manager, so that he could invite the patients to select jobs appropriately rather than take complete control himself, with the patients sitting back passively.

Sometimes a report back to the community in no way reflects the hard work that a group may have put into an attempt to solve a problem. For example, a group was concerned about missing cutlery and needed the community's co-operation to organize a search. The works manager, however, put it differently and said to the community, 'Now, all those who've been flogging knives in the market, please watch out. We are watching you!' By trying to make a joke of it he defeated the group's serious intention that the problem be owned by the whole community. The group took the matter up with him later and pointed out that he was devaluing them and giving the impression that he did not take them or the issue seriously.

The nurse's role in the work group will often be misunderstood. Some patients will expect her to be some kind of therapist and to solve all the group's problems. They will sit back quietly waiting for her to take the lead. When she shows that this is not her task, the group may become angry with her. At some point, the nurse may have opportunity to discuss her role.

For example, a group was cleaning the common room, while a new patient sat down and watched. After a time she said to the nurse, 'Why are you doing all this cleaning? That's all the nurses seem to do here. It's stupid. Anyone could do it.' The nurse asked her what she felt the nurse's work should be. She said, 'You should be talking to us, finding out what our problems are.' The nurse asked her if she thought something could be learned about her problems from the way she was behaving now. She grinned and said, 'You're right. I'm a lazy beggar. Half the time I don't care tuppence about helping anyone else.' She picked up a duster and worked with the group until it had finished.

Work becomes difficult when there is confusion of roles. One group was being heavily challenged by a disturbed member to relieve her distress and explain her behaviour. The nurse could see that the patient was forcing a therapeutic role on the group, which rightly belonged to the doctor. She had to help the group to accept the patient as she was and to show that she, the nurse, recognized that the group could not do much about the patient's personal distress but that she valued what it could offer, by including the patient in the work and helping her to feel she belonged, was needed, and could contribute in a working role.

MEDICAL AND NURSING ROLES

Medical and nursing roles were further clarified and the doctor's therapeutic relationship with the patient better safeguarded during this period of community development. While both work with patients, the doctor uses his psychotherapeutic skills and the nurse her psychosocial skills – different, not confused but complementary,[1] as the above illustration shows. A sharper picture is drawn in the example that follows.

One night some milk bottles were broken and left outside the consulting room of the doctor treating a group of adolescents. A cleaner found the mess next morning, was very cross, did not clean it up but fetched the nurse to see. The nurse reported the event to the community meeting and asked if anyone knew anything. Silence. The two suspects huddled together at the back of the room. Turning to the adolescents as a group the nurse asked again. Another silence. Then discussion began: Should the cleaner come to the meeting and make the protest herself? Should she have left broken glass on the stairs? The doctor would be sure to see it when he came in. Could we deal with this incident in a community meeting or should it be taken up in a treatment session? What if the children slipped and cut their feet? Then the meeting became angry. What were the cleaners here for if they didn't do their job? The doctor should have his nose rubbed in it. The adolescents were always doing things like this; they should be punished.

Eventually the two suspects owned up, adding defiantly that they would not be going to treatment session that day and that they most certainly would not clean up the mess. The nurse offered to help them. Time was running out. Two minutes before the treatment session was due to begin they left the meeting with the nurse, cleaned up the mess just in time, and went in for their session with the others.

The doctor is concerned with the patient's internal world and the therapeutic relationship is private and confidential between the two (or between the doctor and the group of patients, as the case may be). This privacy is threatened whenever the patient causes disturbance in the external world of such a nature that the attention of the community is drawn to the matter. Such behaviour may occur when there is some difficulty in the therapeutic relationship and the patient seeks to bring his problem to other people (in the above example, to the community of staff and patients), hoping for some solution better and more immediate than that provided in the therapeutic relationship. The role of the community is not to usurp the role of the doctor but to deal with the problem realistically in

[1] See also Chapter 6 – Ed.

so far as it affects the relationships and work of the community. The nursing skill lies in helping the community and its individual members to get on with the work and maintain adult roles. When the patient can achieve working and social relationships that do not disturb other people, the nature of his problem in the therapeutic situation is of no concern to the community and the privacy of his communication with the psychotherapist is safeguarded.

CHANGES IN TRAINING

Though the nurse's interest has become increasingly centred on groups and the community, the nursing task remains essentially the same. Thus the basis of nurse training continues to be the understanding of child development.[1] Some changes in the training programme have been made, however.

With mothers and children and, later, complete families in the community, the nurses had more opportunity to observe and work with children and no longer needed to attend the local nursery schools as they had done previously for practical experience and teaching material. Virtually all training could occur in the current situation in the hospital. It became more difficult, however, for new nurses to understand in an emotional sense the child's internal phantasy world. They tended to see only the child or adult patient responding to external and environmental situations.

The first attempt to make up for this deficiency was by observation through a one-way screen into the children's playroom. This proved to be too provocative to the children, their mothers, and the other patients, and to the nurses. Furthermore, the nurses were observing intellectually; their emotional involvement was too superficial to provide the basic learning experience. The attempt was abandoned after six months.

Training continued to be related to a play group held every morning for children under three, with mothers and nurses joining in. Some mothers who could not play with their children found support in this setting. The senior nurse could explain to them and to the junior nurses what the children might be experiencing as shown in their play. Often they seemed to reflect current events that were worrying their mothers.

For example, when a patient, Janet, was admitted to sick bay

[1] See also Chapter 3 – Ed.

immediately on arrival in response to staff anxiety about her emaciated condition, and her care was controlled by the staff, the patients felt that she had been 'banished', and that she was a special patient who got more than her fair share of nursing time and attention. One particular morning at the community meeting, all attempts to discuss the problems she created for other patients and for the nurses were strongly resisted. The fact that she hovered between life and death was denied and the meeting ended without any acknowledgement of anxiety or concern. But in the play group, going on at the same time as the community meeting, the children were demonstrating their anxiety unmistakably. They were busy making Plasticine cakes and feeding them to each other. Then a four-year-old girl, older than the others, told the youngest child to get into bed, she was ill. The little one did so and for a time they all played doctors and nurses. One child came over to the nurse and asked, 'Where *is* sick bay?' At once, a little boy said, 'You die there!' When the nurse explained that Janet was there and that they were worried about her, the little boy chirped up, 'She's going to have a baby.' Group play stopped at this point and the children went back to individual play.

Observation of events such as this helped the nurses to understand more of what might be happening in the community, and something of the child's phantasy life could be caught. But the training problem remained: how to help the nurse to become aware of the child in herself in such a way that she could understand the children and the child in the adult patient without becoming personally disturbed.

The next change was to combine the role of tutor with that of the senior nurse in the medical unit, which, at the time, was primarily interested in mothers and children. All new nurses worked in this unit for their first six months. They could be involved in a continuous situation which provided the basic learning experience, and to which all discussions and explanations could be geared. The tutor, being also the unit's senior nurse, was in close daily contact with the trainees and the unit's doctors, involved in every situation likely to cause stress, and could call conferences and institute administrative and nursing procedures as circumstances demanded.

This arrangement was later extended to other medical units. In the most recent training programme, each new nurse works with a senior nurse, caring for and working with a group of families, adolescents, and single adults, as described earlier in this chapter.

The changes in the training programme reflect medical developments over the years and are designed to balance the kind of nursing required by the medical staff and the training needs of the new nurses.[1] Essentially, it has been found necessary to provide situations for the relief of tension and emotional disturbance arising from disagreements, divided loyalties, and uncertainties in the working area, so that unnecessary strain is not put into the learning-teaching situation. New ideas and new ways of thinking and behaving provide their own emotional consequences and require slow and often painful psychic work for the new nurse.

[1] See also Chapter 3, final paragraph – Ed.

PART IV

Application of Psychosocial Nursing

Editorial Note

The papers in this Part show how some of the concepts and techniques of the psychosocial nursing speciality were brought into the thinking and practice of the nursing profession as a whole.

Doreen Weddell's first two papers concern the education and selection of nurses. She advocates a rearrangement of the training programme to enable the student nurse to begin her training in the place where illness itself begins and is first dealt with, in the patient's own home. Her second paper demonstrates selection as a two-way process and suggests how the procedures employed in the Cassel Hospital could be modified for use in other hospitals.

T. F. Main presents the Cassel selection procedure, perhaps the one routine to remain virtually unchanged since it was instituted in 1946, a fact that testifies to the soundness of the basic planning.

In the following paper, Doreen Weddell gives a succinct explanation of the psycho-analytic concept of object relations and shows how it could be useful to matrons in the selection and training of nursing staff.

Her next paper presents a pattern of ward administration redefining lines of authority and responsibility and avoiding the bewildering array of contacts the patient is required to make. The pattern is worked out in more detail in Eileen Skellern's report of her research on the role of the ward sister. Since their original publication, some of the ideas in these two papers have been modified to become standard nursing practice.

The final paper traces some of the changes in attitudes to hospitals following changes in their function and management, particularly in the United Kingdom, during this century.

21 · *The Education of the Nurse*[1]

Plea for a Particular Experiment

BY DOREEN WEDDELL

Experiments are already being carried out in certain areas of the country with regard to nursing patients in their own homes, particularly children, sometimes old people, and certain medical cases. I should like to see these experiments extended and to suggest a possible way of thinking about training nurses with this approach to the patient as its basis.

Before this can be done, however, there are many questions to be asked and answered, and these require the active interest, co-operation, and leadership of the medical profession; but the nurse, because of her close contact with patients, may be able to point a way in which investigation and experiment might proceed.

HOSPITAL OR DOMICILIARY CARE

As our knowledge of how people come to think, feel, and behave as they do is increased, so does the relationship of one person with another assume greater importance. In recent years attention has been called to the possible deleterious effects of disturbances within the family that result from the enforced separation of one member from another – through wartime evacuation, for example, or through divorce or illness. Children have been shown to be particularly vulnerable in this respect, but many people will agree that adults can also experience upsets of a not dissimilar nature. Is there anything that can be done to reduce such disturbances within a family when illness occurs? What percentage of patients have to be admitted to hospital for purely clinical considerations, not for

[1] Extracts from a paper published in the *Nursing Times*, 16 September 1955.

the doctor's, the pathologist's, or other specialist's convenience, but because the patient really cannot be treated clinically in the home? What percentage of patients could be treated at home if nursing, domestic, and other social help were available? Would there be any difference in the speed and ease of recovery and return to work of the sick person if he were nursed at home and if the family's resources could be augmented by appropriate help from the hospital or local authority? Would he have cost the country more or less? What is the effect likely to be on the national health service budget or on the country's productivity? Is the family in better or worse shape emotionally and economically when the sick member is treated at home rather than in hospital?

There are no easy answers to these questions, for no two families are quite the same and different areas of the country may require different services, but small-scale experiments might give some indication of possible answers. Emphasis on the home would probably mean a reorientation of medical, nursing, and domestic services of the area, with altered roles and relationships of general practitioners, and hospital and local authority staff; the need would be for teams of doctors, medical auxiliaries, nurses, social workers, domestic and other helpers, prepared to give what assistance the family required at the time of illness. Looking after the patient in his own setting might well be found to be not only exacting, but enriching and rewarding in new ways.

DEVISING A RADICAL EXPERIMENT

As far as the nursing profession is concerned, such an approach to the patient might allow for a reorganization of nurse training, to permit the student to begin her experience by working with a senior nurse in a home situation, and to progress in the course of her training to experience in hospitals. This, in turn, might revolutionize the approach to patients in hospitals: one can imagine that certain procedures, tasks, and events in the ward now taken as essential for the wellbeing of patients and staff might at least be questioned in the light of nursing in other situations.

Many people would be involved in any change along the lines indicated, and almost all of them would have doubts and difficulties which would have to be examined. But I should like to see a matron of enthusiasm and vision getting together with her opposite numbers in the district nursing and health visitor fields, along with their respective tutors, to explore how a radically different kind of training within a very limited area could be devised. The help, interest, and vision of the hospital's senior medical staff and the medical officer of health would be needed, as well as the support of the general practitioners of the locality. It is difficult to make a start on implementing any of these ideas because there are so many vested interests, not forgetting those of the family itself, and it is easy to be discouraged before anything tangible is achieved. The experience of those who have already gone some way in the direction of providing the needed services for the patient in the home will be invaluable.

It is probably true that the population falls very broadly into two groups: (*a*) those who prefer not to go to a doctor or a hospital except as a last resort, and (*b*) those who go to one or other member of the health team at the slightest provocation. Over the years this latter group of people has been led to believe that hospitals have 'the magic' and that only in hospital can you get the best treatment, whether this involves having a baby, a dressing for a cut finger, the relief of a pain in the big toe, or, more realistically, a surgical operation. Illness and death are very frightening to most people and to be able to send the patient to hospital is reassuring; yet at the same time relatives are often resentful that they are not considered capable of doing anything for the patient at the moment of crisis. Any experiment along the lines suggested would involve helping the families to use the common sense and skills that they possess, and it would presumably be the task of one member of the therapeutic team to assess the families' capacities and needs and to protect them from an influx of too many helpers.

Assuming, then, that in some parts of the country the trend of the future might be towards treating as many patients as possible in their own homes, could advantage be taken of this for the training of the nurse? Could the student begin her training by looking after patients in their own environment? She would work under a trained nurse, of course, and would need some preliminary instruction, but such a situation, not unlike that of looking after Mum or Dad, or brother or sister, at home, may be nearer to the phantasy of an adolescent as to what nursing is going to be than is the well-ordered and disciplined ward of the hospital, with 'cases' in neat rows of beds. The attraction and the glamour of going to hospital, with its bustle and efficiency, could still be kept, for that could be the next step in the nurse's training.

THE BASIC PATTERN

Could nursing the patient in the home be the basic pattern of nurse training in the future, with experience in hospital in the various specialties as part of the training? The preliminary training schools could prepare students with such knowledge as they would require to make them useful aides to senior nurses looking after patients in their own homes. Short periods in medical, surgical, children's, and psychiatric wards in a large hospital might complete the basic training. The nurse would then have to choose in which specialty she wanted to gain further experience: nursing in the home or nursing in hospital. The whole service to the patient might be carried out from the hospital, at the request of a general practitioner, and a period of working with the hospital team visiting the sick patient in the home and doing the active nursing there would be required before the nurse could hold a supervisory position. Similarly, further experience in all forms of ward care of patients would be necessary before a supervisory position of any kind could be achieved in a hospital. It would be possible to differentiate grades in the specialty a nurse had chosen, for instance, surgical ward nurse, surgical home nurse; medical, psychiatric, or children's ward nurse or home nurse.

Could this approach go any way towards meeting the current problems of the nursing profession (the wastage of students, for instance)? With a shortened basic training the nurse would have an earlier opportunity of finding the right niche so that she could develop her particular interests and skills. Salaries and conditions for the various grades would have to be more or less commensurate, while allowing for as wide a differentiation as possible for special ability.

Any thoughts about the education of the nurse must eventually return to the needs of the patient, and thence to the trends of medicine. The ideas just discussed are thrown out in the hope that they will stimulate further thought, discussion, correspondence, and, eventually, action that will keep the nursing profession not only in line with the needs of the community of today, but also ready for tomorrow.

22 · *A Contribution to Selection Procedures for Nurses*[1]

BY DOREEN WEDDELL

Faced with the task of providing enough nurses, most matrons have become what might be called 'good choosers'. Few find it difficult to choose the best and reject the worst of a group of candidates, but in between come a large number of people with a wide range of assets and capabilities and it is not so easy to decide with any certainty which of them would be suitable for the profession. When someone turns out to be less good than expected, we feel, uncomfortably, that one of the others not chosen might have turned out better after all.

Few hospitals can afford failures. One misfit can cause a situation of increasing stress and difficulty and it is not always the matron who chose her who primarily suffers from the discord. When one nurse leaves out of her particular group, others in the group tend to leave also. The selection of the right person, then, reduces the wastage rate in two ways: first, through the satisfaction of the individual and, second, through her effect on others.

The rather hit-and-miss method of ordinary interviewing often does not tell us enough about the candidate to enable us to make a choice with any degree of certainty. Yet it is proper to consider whether, with the chronic shortage of nurses, it is really practical to introduce a selection system which may appear to reduce the possible number of acceptable candidates. A hospital that takes itself seriously enough to choose its staff carefully, however, not only improves its morale but becomes known for good relationships, which will attract candidates. Unsuitable candidates will be a waste eventually and taking them on, even for a few months, is a poor

[1] Adapted from a paper given at a conference of the Royal College of Nursing, 1950.

policy. It disturbs them and causes trouble for those they work with, thus it is bad both for them and for the hospital. Is it worth taking an inadequate 'pair of hands', bearing in mind the cost in money, time, labour, and discouragement of the girl herself and of her colleagues? Is it not economic to use some of that time, money, and labour to find out more about the candidate before accepting her? As for selecting senior staff, the Working Party Report (Ministry of Health, 1947) recommended 'a new procedure in selecting nurses for senior posts which would ensure that only those who possess the capacity for developing satisfactory human relationships should be appointed'. If this recommendation were implemented, its effect would be seen in some reduction of wastage rates.

To assume that selection of staff will solve all the problems of recruitment and wastage is a magical notion. Unreliable procedures are a danger and we must be prepared to experiment before discarding our present methods.

How, then, can we get to know what kind of person the candidate is, what sorts of relationship she will form, and what use she will make of the experiences she will have in the course of training or working?

Selection procedures such as those used by the War Office Selection Boards in the Second World War are largely concerned with ascertaining interests, aptitudes, and potential capacities, and matching these with the requirements of specific jobs. Nursing, however, does not lend itself to such clear definitions. So many skills and interests go to make the art of nursing that no one particular characteristic is likely to produce the best nurse. Most people involved in experimental schemes of selection will agree that the total personality is more important than any one aptitude.

With increasing emphasis on preventive health and social medicine, it is worth noting that not every one who trains as a nurse needs to be an expert bedside nurse. Florence Nightingale herself said, 'I look forward to the day when all *sick* nurses will be *health* nurses.' The day has yet to come when bedside nursing will be regarded as only one aspect of the total training of the health nurse. Different kinds of people can become satisfactory nurses. A hundred patients might choose a hundred different nurses if each chose the one he liked best.

Perhaps the first point to be made about a selection procedure is that it must be acceptable to everyone concerned. The matron and other selectors must feel easy about the method and it should not be disturbing to the candidate.

THE SELECTION TEAM

Who has the final choice? The only proper answer to this question must be the matron, the nursing head of the hospital and training school. Experts with technical skill can help her by placing before her facts about the candidate which may not emerge at an ordinary interview. She can then make her choice in the light of a variety of objective assessments and not only on the basis of her personal opinion. Some psychologists and psychiatrists, who have special experience in personality assessment and interview techniques, can contribute without interfering with the matron's right to choose the kind of nurse she herself prefers. The traditions of many of our hospitals have been founded successfully on just this kind of personal prejudice. There is no doubt, however, that the service of a trained interviewer is most valuable and it is his or her contribution of objective personality findings that ensures the success of the procedure.

The medical staff, who help to train the nurse and who make ever greater demands on her technical skill, could be asked to assist the matron to choose the kind of nurse they require. The medical examination could be used to provide information about the candidate as a human being as well as to record her physical health.

The people she will be working with could co-operate in the choice of their colleague. It is likely to make for better relationships if the ward sister is involved in the choosing of her own staff nurse. Where wards are organized into units, the ward sisters should have some say in the selection of a new sister. Medical staff could help to choose their ward sisters, and vice versa. When choosing students or deciding if a student should continue after the preliminary training period or the first-year examinations, the matron should act on the advice of the tutors and senior nurses who have been working with her. It is the people in daily contact with the candidate who know most about her. It is not difficult to think of many awkward situations that might have been avoided if the people concerned could have been involved in the selection.

THE CANDIDATE'S PART IN SELECTION

Selection is a two-way process. The candidate should get the feeling that she is having a fair deal, with ample opportunity to ask questions and to see not just the building but something of the life of the hospital community. It is useful to postpone questioning the the candidate about herself until she is satisfied about the people doing the selecting and how far their expectations of her balance her own ideas about what she wants to do. If she feels easy about discussing these things she is likely to be less anxious and more honest during the interview.

The procedure should not be concerned solely with accepting or rejecting. The very method of rejecting requires thought. Facts discovered about the candidate can be used to give constructive help in discussing her future career. One candidate, for example, may be efficient, conscientious, good in emergency, and may enjoy routine work and the satisfaction of technical skills rather than close personal contact with patients. She may not make a good ward sister but might well be advised to consider theatre work.

Every candidate, even the rejected, should be able to feel that applying for the job was worth while. Her belief in her own value should not be impaired by the selection procedure.

PROCEDURE DESIGN

The design to be adopted must be discussed by all those concerned so that their needs and the selection tests are matched. What is being sought in the candidates must be known and agreed to. Certain general qualities such as conscientiousness, optimism, even temper, altruism, will generally be expected. It is not possible, though, to measure or apportion these qualities accurately. The aim can only be to get as full and deep a knowledge of each candidate as possible. The procedure is simply a method of getting it. Candidates who are unimpressive at the interview should have other opportunities to show their assets. It should be possible to recognize those whose qualities are all on the surface and who have little depth to their characters.

Any selection procedure begins with the advertisement, the first sweep of the net, as it were. The quality of the candidates presenting themselves is determined, to some extent, by the quality of the advertisement and this is inevitably a limiting factor in the selection process.

The first part of the procedure, once the candidates have arrived, is best devoted to satisfying their need for information, to showing what is on offer. The second part is concerned with getting information from the candidate and finding out what she has to offer. Such information may be sought by providing situations which allow us to see how the candidate does things, how she gets involved in various activities, and what she feels about them.

If the candidates are invited to spend the whole day in the hospital as a group, they can develop a certain security with each other and face, for better or worse, the day together. The manner of their reception is important. One or two nurses of the candidates' status could welcome them and put them at ease, with tea and about fifteen minutes' talking together.

The candidates need to meet the matron quite soon and to hear from her something about the hospital, especially its people. Some information about the matron herself will help the candidates to decide if she is the kind of person to whom they could be loyal.

During the tour of the hospital, it is useful to introduce some of the many people encountered and to provide opportunity for the candidates to ask questions about the work they do and how they fit into the community.

The second part of the procedure gives the candidate an opportunity to show her assets, capabilities, aims, interests, maturity level, and her emotional response to pleasant and unpleasant events.

Clues to personality can be provided by projection tests which allow the candidate to throw light on different features of herself, such as her response to human distress, her capacity for independent thinking, her sensitivity, the maturity of her social relations. Sometimes these clues are of doubtful significance, but a tentative judgement about the main emotional patterns can usually be made and confirmed or rejected later at the personal interview. Interpretation of the responses to these tests is a matter for the expert: it requires technical understanding of personality development and of the ways in which it can be revealed. Personality handicaps and weaknesses are not important in themselves; it is the manner in which such difficulties are handled that indicates the strength, sensitivity, and resilience of the individual.

A group discussion shows how the candidates manage social situations. They sit in a circle with a staff member who initiates but does not direct the discussion. The setting is a complex one and puts the candidate in a dilemma: she needs to distinguish herself in what she knows to be a test situation, yet she must remain socially acceptable to the others. What is actually said during the discussion is not so much of interest to the observer as how each candidate deals with the situation, the quality of the response she evokes in the group, and the degree of her isolation or participation. Other facts will emerge: the need to dominate or the response to being dominated, the wish to lead and the capacity to be accepted as leader, persistence or submission in the face of argument, reconciliation of opposing viewpoints, tolerance of others, the capacity to disrupt or unite a group and make discussion fruitful. The group situation reveals much that is concealed or hardly apparent at an individual interview.

Individual interviews with a doctor, knowledgeable about personality assessment, and with the matron, provide other opportunities for the candidate to express herself. The doctor will have with him the personality pointers and such other facts as have been already ascertained, and his task will be to synthesize these with what the candidate feels able to tell him about herself. The interview should allay rather than produce anxiety and must end on a note of equality and professional respect.

The matron is concerned primarily with whether or not she personally likes the candidate. She can use the interview for getting to know the candidate and, in the case of senior appointments, her professional capacities. Of all those involved in the selection, the matron is the one person who can be subjective and give her personal opinions and prejudices free expression.

ASSESSMENT

All who have been concerned in the above programme must meet together to pool and discuss their findings – the nurses who received the candidates, the nurse tutors, the psychologist who interpreted the projection tests, the interviewing doctor, the staff member who took the group discussion, with the matron in the chair. A written objective description of their findings for each candidate will be presented. The description should avoid qualitative findings, comments on suitability, and technical jargon. With the information pooled and fully discussed, the matron, having regard to all the selectors' views and the unbiased technical data, can make her final decision in the light of her own interview and personal impressions.

The above is a description of a selection procedure for candidates who are new to the hospital. It is one adapted from that in use at the Cassel Hospital.[1] Where candidates are known, by virtue of having spent their training days or some of their working experience in the hospital, the same principles will operate but the procedure may be different.

Psychological tests can never take the place of the ordinary day-to-day practical experiences of a person's capabilities and relationships. The various people who have worked with the candidate can provide answers to such questions as: How does this person do her job? How does she get on with her colleagues? What kind of response does she evoke in them, and they in her? What use has she made of her experience to date? In short, what kind of person is she?

If a ward sister's post is being filled from the hospital's own staff nurses, the people most likely to provide this information are the ward sisters, perhaps some of the junior staff, and certainly the medical staff they have worked with. Facts, not opinions, are required. But in the final choice, made in the light of these facts, the personal prejudices of the matron can again be allowed to operate.

The procedure described could be adapted for selection to any post in any hospital. The aim is to know as much as possible about the candidate in a limited period of time. The method used to get this information, and the use made of it once obtained, would depend on the needs of the individual hospital and the post it is offering. For example, in choosing a theatre nurse, a manual dexterity test would provide additional evidence on the candidate's capabilities.

People repeat in adult life the behaviour and relationships they experienced as children. Through study of these, it is sometimes possible to indicate broadly how people will react to particular situations and other people.

For example, the keen, efficient person, anxious to please, meticulous in detailed work, who loves law and order and may depend on

[1] See Chapter 23 – Ed.

routine work for her security is excellent provided she knows just what to do and when and where to do it. But if the routine is upset she tends to become anxious and cannot decide between essential tasks and trivial details. Such a person may find it difficult to rise to sudden emergency and when several things happen at once and disrupt the routine she will feel threatened.

There are people who need praise to keep going, particularly from parental or authority figures such as the ward sister, doctor, or matron. Given the praise there is almost no end to the amount of interest they will show, the work they will do. So long as the world is kind and appreciative, they are happy and effective.

Discussion at the selection conference will centre on points such as these. Sometimes it will be possible to predict which situations are likely to be stressful to a particular candidate. Given a knowledge of the demands and satisfaction of the post, and the capabilities of the candidates, it should not prove difficult to decide who will be the best one for it.

In the selection of students, however, it is unlikely that projection tests will give a clear indication of how the young person will develop to maturity. It is, none the less, worth while to discover the quality of the candidate's friendships and interests. Her attitude to and relationship with her parents may indicate how she will respond to the authority and discipline of hospital life.

A detailed psychosomatic history is useful. Sickness and absenteeism may well be reduced through knowledge of the kinds of situation that result in certain illnesses, particularly the minor aches and pains.

In any experimental selection scheme, it is essential to keep adequate records in order to evaluate and improve the procedure. A note of caution should be sounded – no procedure is infallible. None can predict how a candidate will in fact react to hospital life and the work she will do. But just as we would not accept a candidate without a report on her physical health, so it would seem reasonable to ask also for information on her intellectual and emotional make-up. The procedure outlined here is no more than an extension of methods already in wide use. It makes possible more adequate knowledge of a candidate than can be gained from the usual interview. It does not allow for rating a nurse good or bad, but gives the selectors freedom to make a choice about the kind of person they would like to see in a particular job.

To summarize: a selection procedure should aim to acquire facts about an individual's personality that can be placed before the matron, who will then make the final choice, and it should be concerned with the needs of the candidate as well as the needs of the hospital.

23 · *Selection of Nurses*[1]

BY T. F. MAIN

The intensive nursing of patients with neurosis makes considerable demands on the emotional maturity of the nurse. It is no light task to tolerate anxiety which proves overwhelming to patients, to work sympathetically with neurotic people while retaining objectivity, to nurse distress with sensitivity and friendliness but without personal emotional involvement or reactions. Not all nurses befitted by training and personality for other branches of nursing can be expected to meet the demands of neurosis nursing without difficulty. Personal maturity and stability are not universal.

When it was known that the hospital, in addition to having to deal with ordinary problems of turnover and with the problem of selecting nurses for the Cassel Bursaries, was likely, in the measurable future, to increase its total number of nurses, it was decided, in 1946, to institute a system of selection that would permit nursing candidates to reveal their relevant assets and liabilities more fully than they could do at a single short interview, and to employ test procedures that would give in the time available as much knowledge as possible on which to base selection judgement.

It was first necessary to decide what must be sought in the candidate, and it was quickly realized that while it was easy to list desirable qualities (such as conscientiousness, imperturbability, even temper, optimism, altruism, etc.) there was no satisfactory method of testing for these except by extravagant and unvalidated procedures. Even if there were reliable methods of measuring these, it would still be difficult to assess the significance in one candidate of the abundance of one quality and the comparative absence

[1] Reprinted from the Cassel Hospital *Medical and General Reports* for the year ending 31 December 1946, by kind permission of the management committee.

of another – proportionate 'weighting' would not be easy. Moreover, it would be difficult to compare one candidate with another as far as suitability for this work was concerned, even though the scores for the different qualities were known; that is, the performance of the whole candidate could not be reliably deduced from a study of the sum of the parts. In the end it was plain that the personalities of suitable candidates would differ not only widely but legitimately, and that no two good nurses need necessarily be alike. Further, it was plain that the final choice must depend on the supply, and that the most that could be asked of a selection procedure was that it should help in choosing from the candidates who presented themselves those most suitable for the tasks at issue.

It was aimed to get as full and deep a knowledge of each candidate as possible, in order to gain an overall picture of the individual with her total human assets and liabilities, and to approach the candidate with no preconceived ideas of what the role required. After the overall picture had been gained we would ask ourselves: 'How is this candidate likely to perform in this hospital?'

While emotional stability would be sought, it was clear that the test procedure should also reveal something of the variety, the colour and richness, of the personality. High intelligence would not be essential, but if intelligence was below a certain level (IQ 110) the candidate would probably find the work too puzzling unless she had an unusually suitable personality.

Two further considerations then arose about the design of the test procedure. First, it would have to be acceptable and non-traumatic to candidates and should, if possible, be an interesting and rewarding experience in itself. The candidate should get something from, as well as give something to, the selection procedure. Second, it was manifest that the engagement of a nurse is a two-way choice process, and that the nurse's choice of the hospital was as much a matter for care as the hospital's choice of the nurse. If full and detailed information about the nurse was to be asked, she must in return be permitted full and detailed information about the vacant role. If she was to be observed in action, she must also be allowed to observe us in action.

After several experiments during which the more obvious mistakes were made, the following procedure, which represents our current practice, was evolved.[1] It has recognizable limitations but is practicable and very much more satisfactory to the candidates and the hospital than selection by single or multiple interview. The procedure is thorough enough for candidates to feel that they have a real opportunity to show their qualities and that the selectors are interested in them as people and are relatively unprejudiced. (It is important for each candidate to feel that she has as fair a deal as the others. Rejection of the poorer candidates and acceptance of the best are easy and probably rapid under any selection method, but it was decided to give all candidates the full test procedure to avoid the trauma of early rejection.) The procedure is revealing enough to permit selectors to have greater conviction about their final choices than is possible at single or multiple interview methods.

As mentioned above, the best or worst candidates are easy to select, but a large number of candidates are 'doubtfuls', and it is in the sorting of these that the merit of the procedure has been most apparent to us. It gives the candidate who is unimpressive at interview a chance to show hidden capacities, to show what is 'in the back of the shop as well as in the shop window'. It has prevented the candidate whose excellences are only skin deep from accepting an engagement which would be unsatisfying both for her and for us.

APPLICATION FORMS

Applicants are sent a form by post to be completed and returned a week or two before the test procedure proper. This concerns factual information about the candidate and saves time that might otherwise be spent at interview. Details of age, schooling, training, experience, and professional aims are given, and a questionnaire relating to psychosomatic symptoms and general health is included. The names of two referees are asked, and references are followed

[1] The technique described has been evolved and practised at the Cassel Hospital. The selection procedure owes very much to the techniques of the wartime War Office Selection Boards, but, whereas these occupied a testing time of three days, the procedure to be described had to be made capable of fitting into the period 9.30 a.m. to 5 p.m. of one day. Moreover, the difference in social setting and aim involved considerable review of War Office Selection Board practice.

Minor variations of the procedure have been used at different times. Murray's Thematic Apperception Test has sometimes been replaced by Phillipson's Object Relations Test, but the original form has been regularly turned to, and the paper is a reliable account of the selection procedure used at the hospital since 1946.

up by letter. Thus by the day of the test procedure a certain amount is known of the candidate's past professional and health record.

INVITATIONS TO ATTEND

Invitations to attend the test procedure are sent out by the matron who asks candidates to arrive at 9.30 a.m. and to stay until tea-time. Eight candidates are asked for each selection day. The selection team includes a nurse-guide, two psychiatrists, and the matron, who, as head of the hospital nurses, has the benefit of the views of the team and has the final choice.

INTRODUCTION TO THE HOSPITAL AND TO THE SELECTION PROCEDURE (9.30–11 a.m.)

The candidates are received in the staff common room by the matron and a sister (who is to be their guide) and are introduced to each other over a cup of tea. Conversation is general and informal and this period until 10 a.m. is used to set the candidates at their ease and to permit them to take bearings of their surroundings, of their guide, and of the matron. Towards ten o'clock the matron makes a few remarks about the hospital and its general purpose, and tells the candidates that the first part of the morning will be spent in letting them learn about us and that after 11 a.m. we shall learn something about them. The candidates are then handed over to the nurse-guide who takes them on a tour of the hospital, explaining its work from a nurse's point of view and soliciting and answering questions. The whole hospital is visited and particular attention is paid to those aspects involving nursing activities. On the way round, the guide introduces the eight candidates to any hospital workers met, nurses, doctors, and administrators. The candidates share some degree of security by being in a group, and this and the informal nature of the tour encourage free discussion, an exchange of views on the people and things met. At 10.45 a.m. the candidates return to the staff common room where they may move among and talk to the rest of the staff, doctors, nurses, and administrators, at morning coffee. They have at this stage entered into the staff atmosphere as participants and have the chance of summing up the hospital staff. It is a common remark from candidates that this part of the procedure gives them the 'feel' of the hospital, and that living for even so short a time in the hospital atmosphere they are able to clarify their expectations and match them with the real opportunities (or lack of them) that the hospital offers. At 11 a.m. their guide collects them and conducts them to the test room. She then explains the programme for the rest of the day and they begin the first of the written tests.

PROJECTION TESTS

These written tests aim at providing the candidates with opportunities to respond, in their own characteristic ways, to the same evocative emotional stimuli. By the nature of the responses each candidate reveals something of her habitual emotional patterns and ways of feeling. The tests provide, in fact, clues to the personality. Sometimes these clues have a doubtful significance, but at other times permit tentative judgement about the main emotional patterns, which can be confirmed or rejected later at interview. The interpretation of the responses is a skilled matter needing some understanding of personality development, and the ways in which personality reveals itself. The projection tests are therefore examined by a psychiatrist, who writes a short note on the significant trends revealed by each candidate. This note acts as a 'personality pointer' for the subsequent psychiatric interview.

The tests are administered to the group in a small room, with the candidates seated at desks arranged in a semicircle around their guide, who acts as tester. Four tests are used, as described below.

Thematic Apperception Test (11–11.45 a.m.)

Eight of Murray's original cards are used in constant order. Each card is held up for two minutes, after which the candidate is given three minutes in which to write an account of what is portrayed in the picture. Each picture may be construed in various ways but the nature of the response reveals something of the candidate's prevailing attitude towards people and situations. The test gives the candidate the opportunity to project herself into the situation shown in the pictures and, by her response, to manifest the subtleties of feeling and attitude that are not quickly discernible at ordinary interview. It is not possible to regard the response to any one picture as pathognominic, and indeed the trends that emerge from all eight responses need confirmation from other tests or further elucidation at interview. The amount any one test reveals varies with the candidate, but, taken in conjunction with other tests, the Thematic Apperception findings are one more brick in the construction of the total personality picture.

Word Association Test (11.45–12 a.m.)

This is a modification of Jung's original test. A card on which is printed a stimulus word is held up before the candidates who are asked to write a sentence containing that word. The candidate is given fifteen seconds in which to be ready for the next card. There are sixty-five cards. The words have been chosen for their capacity to evoke significant responses and the list includes words which allow the candidate to throw light upon different features in her make-up, such as her prevailing moods and attitudes, rigidity or elasticity of character, nature and degree of altruism, habitual methods of handling pleasant and unpleasant events, quality of response to human distress, maturity of social relations, capacity for independent thinking, points of personal sensitiveness or uneasiness. The test is not quantitatively scored but a qualitative interpretation is made and the emerging personality themes are noted, so that they may be clarified later at interview.

Self-descriptions (12–12.15 p.m.)

Each candidate is asked to write a short description of herself as a person. It will be realized that the descriptions given by no means represent objective truth but are useful indicators of how the candidate regards herself. Her scales of human values are often revealed in the criticisms or satisfactions she apportions to various features of her make-up, and her ability to be frank, her capacity for insight, and her degree of acceptance of her own human failings may sometimes be made plain; other attitudes towards herself ranging from satisfaction to vanity and from modesty to inferiority feelings are sometimes shown with remarkable vividness. The self-description is not always revealing, but it may manifest with sureness some of the candidate's qualities, and, if cautiously interpreted, sometimes has great value.

At first self-descriptions were obtained by the use of two questions: 'Describe yourself as a good friend would see you'; 'Describe yourself as a hostile critic would see you.' In these forms, self-description was more revealing, but the questions allowed the candidates little room for protective evasion and proved to be disturbing to them. The self-description now used is more acceptable to candidates, and is still of value.

Significant moment

At first candidates were asked to describe the best and then the worst moments in their lives, but these two questions were somewhat puzzling and rather too intimate to be easily accepted. The candidate is now asked to describe in two minutes the most exciting moment of her life.

Again, the test may or may not be revealing and certain responses have only a limited significance, whereas others reveal important trends. Optimism or pessimism, major fears or hopes, childishness or maturity of outlook, altruism or egocentricity, together with points of mental or physical satisfactions, are some of the features that may be revealed in the responses. None of these by itself is considered to be indicative but, when fitted into the other test findings, each helps the selectors to build up a picture of the personality under scrutiny.

Conclusions about projection tests

Taken as a whole the projection tests are a most valuable part of the procedure. At times they reveal quickly and unmistakably the positive and negative qualities possessed by the candidate; at others the findings are indeterminate and need further pursuit at interview. Usually the projection tests reveal to the selectors the main patterns of character development and distinguish the colourful from the colourless individual and the mature from the immature (these being relative terms). It is to be recognized that personality handicaps and weaknesses are not *by themselves* important. Rather, the manner in which the difficulties are handled is important in promoting or handicapping strength, sensitiveness, and resilience in an individual, and it is by indicating the 'character defences' that the tests probably have the greatest value. It is important to interpret the projection tests with objectivity and caution and to be sure that glimpses of the obvious do not prevent search for the richness that comes from finer subtleties.

One psychiatrist interprets all the projection tests. No score is given for any test but each candidate's series is carefully reviewed and the emergent themes are noted by cross-checking the various responses of the candidate. The psychiatrist is then able to write notes about the trends that recur and persist throughout the many responses under review, and to write in ordinary English a description of the candidate as a human being.

INTELLIGENCE TEST (12.15–1 p.m.)

This is introduced to candidates as a test of the 'capacity to learn'. Because of the short time available, a rapid and yet fairly reliable group test had to be chosen. Raven's Progressive Matrices was found to be too well known (especially to ex-service nurses) and the Shortened Wechsler is now in use. Most qualified nurses have no difficulty in satisfying the minimum standard required (IQ 110) and if the test procedure had to be shortened the intelligence test would be the first to go. Given the minimum level of intelligence asked, the suitability of candidates for neurosis nursing depends decidedly more on personality than on high intelligence. Nevertheless the test is useful not only to exclude the occasional low-scorers, but to identify those in whom a particular intelligence level helps to explain certain features of personality. Caution about interpreting low IQs has paid: twice a low score was explained by fatigue from all-night duty or an all-night train journey, once by a severe cold, and twice by general worry.

LUNCH (1–2 p.m.)

The lunch hour is used to permit the candidates further opportunities for seeing something of the hospital. As participant members of the hospital community they get their food at the cafeteria and are free to sit where they want to at small tables by themselves, with staff, or with patients. After lunch, tea in the staff common room permits the candidates further participation in ordinary conversation with hospital staff, while affording them the shared shelter of their own group. They are treated with informality, not as guests, but as potential future staff members. The staff are accustomed to have visitors in the common room and do not react specially to the candidates. An ordinary, easy behaviour sample is thus presented for assimilation by the candidates, who are free to talk and observe at will.

INDIVIDUAL INTERVIEWS (2–3.30 p.m.)

At two o'clock the staff common room empties and the afternoon programme is explained to the candidates. The psychiatric interview lasts ten to forty minutes and two psychiatrists are available, each seeing four candidates. Concurrently with the psychiatric interviews, the matron interviews each candidate for a quarter of an hour. The nurse-guide conducts the candidates to and from interviews, and gossips with them, answering questions and giving information about the nurse's work in the hospital. In the security of their group, candidates are now talking freely, usually about the test procedure, and sharing, from common experience acquired, a sense of identity.

Psychiatrist's interview

The psychiatrist is now in possession of the candidate's completed application form, giving details of schooling, health, family situation, and career information, together with the IQ, and the summary of the candidate's 'personality pointers' as revealed by the projection tests. Certain interviewing principles need mention, for a selection interview differs considerably from a clinical interview. The task is not to seek out or diagnose emotional disturbance but to gather significant material and clarify the issues already raised in the written tests, and to acquire further positive and negative information. The psychiatrist's knowledge of mental mechanisms and personality growth helps him to synthesize information thus far gathered into a whole, where the basic drives and their habitual methods of operating are understood. The interview must protect the candidate from trauma and must resolve rather than produce anxieties. The candidate's personality is accorded full respect, and by offering sincerity in discussion the psychiatrist provides a basis for easy relationship in which the candidate is given full freedom to tell more about herself if she wants to. Leading or abrupt questions are avoided and the interview is begun by using the written information set out by the candidate as an opening topic. Once the candidate feels easy enough to talk about herself, the psychiatrist may invite her comment on matters which may throw light on the trends already suggested by the personality pointers. The test procedure having been so far friendly and purposive, most candidates want to tell something more about themselves and, where sufficient time is given for 'warming up', the candidates may discuss readily the stress points within themselves and their points of view about themselves. The psychiatrist must judge when or if he may ask for further information. By now most candidates, assured of the preservation of their self-esteem, may ask for the psychiatrist's opinion and even for his advice. Towards the end of the interview the psychiatrist leads the candidate back to more general topics of conversation and, so to speak, reinstates the candidate in her role of an independent professional woman, so the interview ends on a note of professional respect and equality.

Following the interview the psychiatrist writes an objective description of the personality as a whole. This description is written in ordinary English with conscious objectivity and the avoidance of condemnation or approbation.

Matron's interview

Here objectivity is not sought. The other members of the test team have the task of avoiding prejudice and seeking knowledge. The matron, as head of the nursing service, must, however, like the candidate personally if the engagement is to be satisfactory, and she uses the fifteen-minute interview to find out more about the candidate in ordinary terms of human behaviour and professional interests and capacities, and forms her own conclusions. She is the one member of the team in whom objectivity is not imperative, and her personal feelings about the candidate are given due status.

GROUP DISCUSSION (3.30–4.30 p.m.)

Eight candidates now assemble in a seated circle together with the psychiatrist,[1] who initiates a group discussion. The psychiatrist after the first few minutes does not lead the discussion; rather, he helps it to develop until he is able to take up his task of observing the performance of the candidates in this group situation.

The social situation is, of course, a complex one. Each candidate has a need for competitive distinction in the presence of the psychiatrist and yet has to remain socially acceptable to the other candidates. Her method of solving this dilemma situation, through discussion, is under review by the observer who notes the quality

[1] The group discussion is now taken by a nurse, a practice first begun a few years after this report was published – Ed.

of the response each candidate evokes from the rest of the group, and her degree of social isolation or participation. Group discussion is by no means a simple affair and much information can be gathered from it. The need to dominate and the response to being dominated, the wish to lead and the capacity to be accepted as a leader, persistence or submission in the face of arguments, the reconciliation of opposing viewpoints, tolerance for another's points of view, the capacity to disrupt or set the group at odds, to unite the group and make discussion fruitful, are some of the things about a candidate that may be revealed during the discussion.

Towards the end of the period, the psychiatrist again takes a more active role, resolving opposing views and tying together the threads of a discussion, easing by comment and review any feelings that may have been engaged during the session.

It is in the field of human relations that the neurosis nurse is to work and it is of particular importance to be able to assess her capacity to form easy, rewarding, or reciprocal relations with others. In the group situation, feeling and attitudes may be revealed which are concealed or hardly apparent at individual interview. The candidate is seen, so to speak, in social action.

TEA AND CRITICISM (4.30 p.m.)

The candidates having been in the hospital community first as visitors, then as participants, and then under scrutiny, it is regarded as important that they should now be reinstated as professional women and be helped to recover their self-sufficiency as individuals with interests outside the hospital. Tea is taken with the matron, who initiates conversation on the level of professional gossip between nurses. The sealing off of the test situations and the restoration of professional self-respect are aimed at, and an opportunity is given to the nurses to criticize the procedure.

Talk about the procedure itself is useful for two main reasons. First, it permits the nurses to talk out doubts which may have been aroused by any part of the test procedure, and to criticize it in whole or in part. This helps in the restoration of self-respect and gives a chance to relieve disturbed feelings. Second, valuable suggestions have been given by candidates about the difficulty or anxiety caused by various parts of the test procedure. In the light of these comments we have discarded those portions of our original plan which were found to cause upset, and have replaced them by procedures which are more acceptable. The candidates' criticisms and suggestions have been helpful and instructive almost without exception, but the most common response to the invitation to say what they think of the test procedure is that it is a rewarding and enjoyable experience for its own sake. Some nurses have said that, even if no engagement results, they still consider the day to have been worth while because of its sheer interest. Others have learned from the day that the posts are not wholly suitable to their particular qualities, and are ready to say so; and yet others are more sure of their wish to work at the hospital. The most common remark is that the test is thorough and gives every candidate a fair chance.

One candidate, unsuitable on other grounds, has been resentful of the whole procedure. A few candidates have disclosed that they themselves were suffering from some emotional upset which they had (wrongly) hoped to solve by taking up psychological nursing, and are grateful for the advice they have been given at the interview.

FINAL CONFERENCE

After each day's testing, while impressions are still fresh, a short conference of the selection team is held, where each candidate's suitability for the nurse's role is discussed. The written tests, the psychiatric interview, the matron's interview, and the group discussion have produced information which is now pooled. Discussion is full and free, and the matron, having the benefit of the views aired and in the light of her own interview, discusses all findings with the selectors and, aided by them, makes her final choices. Technical support or argument is encouraged so that the final decision reached may be taken in the light of all the facts. Common agreement is usually reached in discussion but the final decision is left to the matron.

RATING

Candidates are rated on a five-point scale with the following meanings:

(1) outstandingly suitable
(2) above average

(3) average
(4) below average
(5) outstandingly unsuitable.

It need hardly be mentioned that there are few candidates classed as (1) or (5), and half the candidates obtain the rating (3).

CONCLUSIONS

The test procedure outlined above is workable and valuable both for the candidates and for the hospital. The time spent in choosing a nurse is justified by the absence of subsequent wastage. The letters of thanks received from the candidates suggest that the procedure is usually acceptable to nurses whether they are subsequently engaged or not.

In common with other selection methods, no knowledge is obtained of how many suitable candidates have been rejected. In general, the predictions of performance have been accurate.

24 · *Some Aspects of Personality Development*

BY DOREEN WEDDELL[1]

How do we come to be the kind of people we are, individually so different, yet with some fairly well-defined characteristics? As far as we know, it is not just a matter of genetic, constitutional factors, but an interaction between these and our environmental, cultural, and emotional experiences, the accompanying phantasies and defensive measures we develop to protect ourselves from psychic pain. There would seem to be a kind of internal, dynamic conjugation of experiences, some gradually built into an integrated part of our personality, some separate and unavailable aspects of ourselves, which, together with our unconscious phantasies, may distort our picture of the external world. There are always some aspects of our essential self of which we are only dimly or not at all aware. There also seems to be a strong tendency to repeat various early experiences at intervals throughout life.

The particular aspects of personality development which I believe may be useful for us to think about in relation to the work of matrons are those of object relations.

When we are selecting a candidate for a position or a student for training, we want to know what kind of person we are meeting, how she relates to us and other people; that is, her object relationships in the external world. But her internal world, her relationship with internal parents and family, will colour her perception of the external world.

Let us, therefore, go back to infancy and trace very briefly how a baby begins to relate to his mother, the outside world, his body,

[1] This chapter is based on a paper given to the annual general meeting of The Association of Hospital Matrons, 1955, rewritten for this publication. The theoretical background comes from the work of S. Freud, M. Klein, R. Money-Kyrle, D. Meltzer, W. R. Bion, and H. Segal, in so far as I understand it.

and his developing self. Traces of these early relationships, emotions, and phantasies remain with us all our lives and are the basis of what we call personality.

At first, the infant relates to his mother primarily through his mouth, although smell, skin, fingers, ears, eyes, toes, musculature, genitals, and excretions are important at particular times. Primitive emotions of aggression, envy, jealousy, will affect the infant's recognition of what is being done to him and what he is doing to his mother. As we know, it takes quite a long time for the baby to distinguish himself from his mother's breast, to recognize his mother's face as something apart from himself and his body as different from hers. (Some people may never achieve this successfully and continue throughout life to be confused between internal and external, phantasy and reality.)

The mouth experiences of the infant, if mainly satisfactory, not too exciting or frustrating, will help him to feel his mother to be a satisfying, relieving, and helpful person. When she frustrates, as inevitably she must, she is felt to be unsatisfactory, unpleasant, and unhelpful. The baby begins to equate the first experiences of feeding, bathing, being held, with a good, relieving mother when the experiences are pleasurable and with a bad, hated mother if they are not. The good mother he wants to keep, the bad mother he wants to be rid of, and may feel he is expelling her out of himself in his excretions. The hated mother may then become equated with painful defecations and black moods. Later, the hated mother may be felt as the 'witch' mother, the sexual mother who deserts him for father.[1] Once father is let in, then in phantasy there is a new baby, brothers and sisters, and all are hated because they are felt to be the cause of the mother's desertion. The infant is jealous of them because they are felt to be getting what he wants.

At this stage, he does not want to share and his phantasies are possessive, ruthless, and greedy. His weapons are his screams, scratching fingers, kicking feet, biting teeth, piercing genitals, burning urine and spit, exploding faeces and poisonous flatus. In reality, the weapons are feeble; in phantasy, they are felt to be violent and destructive. At a later stage, the same organs and bodily products can be used to express affection, and the withdrawal of love, by baby or mother, comes to be felt as the most dangerous situation.

[1] See also Chapter 15 – Ed.

The mother's response to the infant will depend on her own internal objects and phantasies and on the extent to which she feels supported, internally and externally, by husband, family, and environment.

For future development, much will depend on the capacity of the infant to introject and preserve an internal (breast-mother-parental) object felt to be strong, relieving, and creative, which will protect him from other objects confused with parts of himself, which are felt to be cruel, threatening, and destructive. The strength and beauty of the internal object can further trust, optimism, and generosity, but if such an object is not satisfactorily established internally, suspicion, spite, and pessimism may ensue.

Once the internal object is felt to be valuable, the wish to spare and protect it can begin to grow. In turn, this will affect the infant's response to inevitable frustration and deprivation, but the loss of the breast or bottle at the time of weaning is bound to be felt as the loss of the only object that can protect him from his persecutors. If he has already been able to recognize that the breast belongs to his mother, and if his trust in her is fairly secure, the external world can be felt as interesting and weaning can have its compensations, with pleasure and excitement in testing, exploring, and mastering new foods and ways of eating.

Weaning is a time of crisis in the infant's developing capacity to be concerned for someone other than himself. When all goes well, he can begin to feel sorrow for his attacks on the loved and valued object. As weaning progresses, something akin to sadness develops, the beginnings of mourning for a lost, valued object. In sparing his mother, and out of concern for her, he finds he can give up the valued object externally while, through the process of mourning, it becomes established as an object in his internal world. This process of external loss, mourning, and internalization will be repeated in some measure at each stage of development as he comes to give up other childhood pleasures.

Some babies turn against the breast at this time and seem to wean themselves. Subsequently, they acquire a brittle kind of independence and competitiveness. Other babies seem to find closeness difficult from a very early age and soon take to the spoon and high chair. But they also make it plain that they wish to be loved, even if they cannot quite allow themselves to be cuddled. They want to be independent, yet always have to go back to what they could not apparently enjoy earlier on. They continue to have a regressive, babyish phase whenever a new step in development has to be taken.

The weaning situation is the foundation of the capacity to tolerate change. Something of the first emotional experiences and responses is repeated whenever adjustments to change are required. It continues throughout life and is experienced by everyone.

With the increasing ability for muscular control, the child begins to play, walk, talk, and use his pot on the right occasions.

In play he may feel he is putting together and restoring what, in phantasy, he has destroyed internally. He feels that he, like his parents, can make babies. There are excited 'I can do it myself' moods. When failure follows, inevitable when the phantasy is an omnipotent one, there can be collapse with a kind of despair arising from the competitiveness in the wish to repair and restore. When this is insufficiently distinguished from aggression, there may be difficulty in sustaining effort and ambition later in life.

In this period, the child's developing differentiation of himself from his parents is important for later judgements about the value of his products and his capacity to do good work. The child discovers that his mother values his bodily products only at certain times and when put in certain places. This discovery will not be too disturbing when trust in the mother has been established. But when there is hatred, rebellion, and suspicion, difficulties may ensue. The child may become particularly sensitive to criticism and, later in life, problems may arise in evaluating his work in relation to that of other people. If a placatory relationship with a persecuting object occurs, there is danger of a kind of enslavement, giving rise to subterfuge, trickery, and subsequent insincere and unreliable relationships.

The child's growing capacity to distinguish between good and bad at this time is important, for when he knows what is bad and who is the enemy, he has a direct outlet for his aggression; concomitantly, there can be increasing admiration for what is loving, restoring, creative, and, therefore, felt to be good. As he begins to recognize the authority of the parents and his dependence, so the distinctions between big and little, masculine and feminine, child and adult, emerge. The struggle then centres on what aspects of care the child can take over for himself and what still has to be exercised by the parents on his behalf until he can take over the parental role himself. How far this is successful at any one stage of development will, again, primarily depend on the strength and understanding of his internal objects. Relics of this struggle continue to be seen in adulthood over questions about what 'they', the 'authorities', should or should not be doing.

During this period another child may be born, providing further opportunities for clarification between the babies inside the mother and the outside babies – the brothers and sisters. The child's capacity to tolerate this event will also depend on what kind of identification he can make with his parents. If, to some extent, he has relinquished his possessive relationship with his mother to allow for developing interest in other people and things, he may be able to equate his own interests and pleasures with those of his parents. If he still feels the need for exclusive possession of the mother, the inevitable rivalry and jealousy may assume major proportions. He may turn against his mother, or may want to become the baby himself. The new baby may have to be protected from his wish to murder it.

Developing relationships with brothers and sisters set the pattern for his future relationships with other children and, later, for his adult perceptions of people older and younger than himself. Good or bad parts of the self may be invested in other children, which, later on, will contribute to the formation of teams, secret societies, and gangs at school, and of clubs, associations, and political parties in adult life.

During the three- to five-year-old period of intense emotional relationships with parents, the child begins to distinguish his wishes from those of his parents and may address himself in their voice over matters of obvious conflict. He will also be heard saying, 'I'm going to marry Mummy', or 'Daddy', as the case may be. 'I wish you would die' may be followed shortly by a hug and kiss to make it up.

As the little boy begins to be the 'man about the house' and to 'go off to work', and the little girl feels like mother with her dolls and pram and helping in the kitchen, both children will want to have babies and are envious of each other's differences. An introjective identification with the parent of the same sex, while maintaining love for the other parent, sets a reasonably good outlook for the future. Sometimes, however, the child wants to 'step into the parents' shoes', a kind of stealing of the role of parent. When this predominates, there is personality impoverishment and instability.[1]

Identification with the bad object may also occur; being the black sheep of the family may be another way of triumphing over the parents and brings its own personality and social consequences.

The child's picture of the parents' sexual relationship will be distorted by his infantile phantasies of cruel attacks; these may continue to be repeated in some of his masturbatory activities. Disturbances in the capacity to enjoy mature adult sexual relationships later in life may derive from the intrusion of these primitive phantasies.

The child's readiness for school will depend on how far his internal family has been satisfactorily established. When there is inadequate differentiation between the internal and external worlds, child and adult, school may be experienced as a persecutory and cruel place, and this will interfere with his capacity to learn.

As he develops relationships with other children, the willingness to protect his family from the criticism and ridicule of other children will be important in the growth of his ability to appreciate the value of various loyalties.

During school days up to the age of puberty, the intensity of the relationship with parents is subsiding and there is increasing opportunity for new identifications and investment of interest and concern, as he sees himself in the context of his family in relation to the community.

Puberty and adolescence bring another chance to work over afresh some of the early emotional and physical responses to parents and environment. Exciting and violent sexual urges come to the fore. This time the youngster has the physical strength and capacity to inflict damage on himself and his objects, if his infantile phantasies are transformed into action in the external world. The outcome of the struggle for control will again depend on how far firm and receptive parental figures can be internalized under the influence of love, care, and concern. When the need for control is directed mainly at internal and external objects, a somewhat rigid personality is likely to result. When supporting, helpful internal

[1] See the example of James, Chapter 18, p. 174 – Ed.

parents are not well established, emotional and physical instability is likely to continue.

The apparent arrogance of the adolescent is part of reality-testing – necessary if childhood illusions and idealizations of self and object are, to some extent at least, given up. As the adolescent achieves a differentiation from his parents and becomes capable of assuming adult roles in relation to his family and the community, the need for a corresponding dependence on internal objects can be recognized. In all the upheaval of this period, there is a continuing sophistication of the categories of thought, with growing distinction between what is valuable, emotionally, physically, intellectually, aesthetically, and culturally, and what is damaging and destructive. Thus develops his particular perception of what may be good or bad, right or wrong.

The capacity to 'feel with other people' would seem to derive from the internalization of a receptive breast-mother-parental object, able to receive experiences and return them in a more understandable form. This appears to be the basis of empathy, which has to be distinguished from the 'getting into someone else's place' referred to earlier.

Throughout life, unwanted emotions, impulses, phantasies, and aspects of the self may be externalized and seen as if they were in other people. While this splitting and idealization partly protect the good internal objects, some aspects of the good self and good impulses are lost along with the rejected parts felt to be bad. An example of this situation may be seen in families in which one or other member often seems to be ill or in trouble, depending on who becomes the repository of the other members' projections.

When there is 'dis-ease' in the psychic family, through the splitting and undermining of internal relationships, the pain and distress may be felt as if coming from a bodily organ. Sometimes physical illness can appear to be a solution to psychic conflict. A particular organ may be chosen for the expression of this kind of 'body language' and some people show clear patterns of physical illness that can be linked with the recurrence of specially disturbing emotional experiences.

To summarize briefly: the pattern of our relationships with people, things, and events, and the categories of our thought about them, develop during the first five or six years of life, but within this pattern there is constant change in our internal world as it is impinged on by internal and external events. Our perception of the external world is similarly affected by the stability or otherwise of our internal family and relationships with various parts of ourselves. Some of us may be mainly optimistic, others are rather pessimistic; but, by and large, ordinary ambitions and pleasures, inevitable upsets, partings, disappointments, will evoke anger, sorrow, love, hate, and jealousy without overwhelming devastations or exultation.

Some people may remain mainly suspicious, critical, demanding, or indifferent. Others may have become so controlling of internal objects that they begrudge the expenditure of emotion, interest, or concern for people in the external world.

A reasonably stable and productive personality seems to be based on an internal world in which the parental object is allowed freedom to be restorative and creative without undue interference from split-off, disowned, infantile parts of the self, or from unconscious, aggressive, envious phantasies. The degree of this emotional freedom will affect the individual's ability to enjoy, adjust to, and be enriched by new experiences.

In what ways can these ideas be of help to matrons in their daily work? Let us explore a few areas as we think about problems familiar to us all.

SELECTION OF STUDENTS[1]

It is not easy to predict how a student, probably still adolescent, will develop during training. But if her capacity to establish satisfactory object relationships is studied, it may be possible to recognize some of the difficulties she might have with senior staff, colleagues, and ward work. The way in which she has previously dealt with events that are exciting and upsetting, such as births, funerals, weddings, parties, partings, and loss, may give some indication of her possible responses to occasions that could have similar significance for her.

If she tends to respond to upset with physical illness, even of a minor nature, the danger may lie in the attraction to her of the reversal of roles in which she becomes the patient (baby), relinquishing responsibility for developing the more adult role of nurse (mother).

[1] See also Chapter 22 – Ed.

Throughout life, some people tend to think in rather concrete terms and respond to suggestions as if they were orders. They may be inclined to put ideas into action before the processes of thought have had time to develop into a 'thinking about' the situation and thus before the action can be modified appropriately to the occasion. Some assessment of how far the student can think through a situation before taking action may be useful.

TRAINING

We accept young people in late adolescence, who are still in a state of sexual unrest and emotional disorganization, as they search for an identity and internal stability. We ask them to face inevitably disturbing situations – death, nakedness, wounded flesh, patients in pain and fear, relatives anxious and unhappy. If the student is to remain sensitive and free inside herself, she needs opportunity to verbalize to some extent the emotional impact of such experiences. If this is not available, there is no model for her to use when she meets patients with similar needs. She may lose some of her concern for other people's feelings and anxieties, if her own have to be denied. When a senior nurse can allow her to share her feelings, without her right to privacy being invaded, a model may be developed so that in her relationships with patients, without encroaching on their right to privacy, she need not be afraid to speak of anxieties, when the occasion seems to indicate it could be helpful.

The student's need to express feelings and ideas can be canalized into the teaching situation. Where discussion is encouraged, in ward and classroom, the student can become increasingly free to speak of the impact on her of people and procedures. She can learn, through verbalizing, what is difficult and painful. Sharing good and bad experiences with others will help her to retain her sensitivity and improve her tolerance for others' difficulties as well as her own. Sometimes the ward teacher, in providing occasions for relief, has to do no more than be there and listen, perhaps commenting from her own experiences of similar occasions. Detailed verbal reports of ward events, including the nurse's feelings, can be used as part of teaching-reporting, and can also be a useful guide to the ward sister in assessing the dynamics of the ward situation at any given moment.

WASTAGE

Some students will inevitably leave training. It will be part of the exploration of their role in the external world, a testing of reality against the phantasy of themselves as the helpful, relieving mother of infancy.

But I think that some other students leave because of the rigidity of our system of training which does not allow for individual differences in the time that may be required to adapt to change. We have seen the importance of how the infant adapts to weaning, the kinds of problem he has in giving up previously desired experiences and adjusting to new people and things. Babies respond differently and take varying periods of time to come to terms with essential changes. So, inevitably, students require different lengths of time in any one learning situation. Each change – from ward to ward, classroom to ward, hospital to hospital – means parting with known relationships and an emotional reinvestment in new people, which affects the learning potential.

As we have seen, enrichment of personality comes from the number and variety of introjective identifications and the capacity for mourning, from which develops the appreciation of beauty, strength, knowledge, and generosity. Something of this can be expected to be part of the student's experience in training and will occur in relation to people – the ward team and patients – and to ideas, as infantile phantasies are tested against the reality presented in the working-teaching situation. For such internal adjustment to be accomplished successfully, a reasonably stable external situation is required and is not always possible with our present method of training.

In the long term, a more satisfactory basic nurse training might come from developing the student's capacity to work in a stable staff team in relation to a group of patients. The patients would change but the team would remain intact, in so far as holidays or imponderables would allow. If it was considered necessary for the student to gain experience in particular departments of the hospital, the team could be moved, thus continuing to provide a relatively stable environment within which learning could occur. It is possible that this method of training could also be of benefit to patients. The student might find such a method more rewarding, as well as less stressful, than working for short periods with a variety of doctors, sisters, and patients with specific illnesses, as in the present system.

SELECTION OF SENIOR STAFF[1]

Differing personalities both choose and make best use of roles commensurate with their personality structure. Assessing the kind of relationship an unknown person will develop with known people is not easy, but we know that patterns tend to be repeated, so that some knowledge of what situations and people the candidate has found difficult or enjoyable may help.

In the choosing of a ward sister, for example, the question of how the candidate deals with depression, her own and other people's, will be important. The nurse who has to deny the work of mourning, essential for emotional recovery, is unlikely to be helpful to patients or to provide a model for staff in this respect. 'Jollying' people along may be useful in the later stages of severe illness, if it is also appreciated that the patient needs periods of quiet withdrawal for the private work of mourning in the restoration of internal objects. Ward sisters who can recognize and make provision for such occasions as part of their nursing skill are likely to be much valued.

The ability to recognize the projection of good and bad objects on to people and situations in the working sphere is also required of senior nurses. Patients may tend to see medical and nursing staff as parental figures rather than as individuals in their own right, and will respond to them according to their own patterns of object relationships. Some will see the staff as mainly helpful people, whereas others will be suspicious and see them as threatening, persecutory figures who have to be fought or placated. The doctor may become the good object and the nurse the bad one, or vice versa.

Similarly, the nurse's perception of her patient, of the doctor, the ward sister, the matron, her colleagues, and others, will be affected by the phantasies, memories, and expectations belonging to family situations of the past, now represented in her internal world and colouring current likes and dislikes, loves and hates.

Sometimes a patient, nurse, doctor, or administrator may become the bad object and be blamed for what is felt to be wrong in the ward, department, or hospital. The senior nurse's awareness of

[1] See also Chapter 22 – Ed.

and ability to deal with such feelings and situations could be important for success in her career.

Nurses responsible for wards, departments, or hospitals may need to understand the dynamics of group situations, rather than the personal problems of the people with whom they work. Who is fighting with whom? Who is undermining whom? Who is being blamed? Who is idealized? Who is usurping whose role or wanting to? These are the questions the nurse in charge could think about and verbalize in seeking to reduce tension, illness, and wastage of staff.

It is not easy to maintain adult roles and responsibilities in the work situation against the subversive incursions of the infantile wish to reduce parental figures to helpless incompetence, and the ward, department, or hospital to a nursery-like state of bickering rivalries. If high morale is to be achieved, the pitfalls of idealization, accompanied by denigration of other people's efforts, need to be heeded.

Understanding a little of how we come to be the kind of people we are is only the first step towards further insight into how groups feel and behave within themselves and towards other groups. This could be the aim for those of us who want to improve skill and reduce stress in any area of our work.

25 · *Human Relations in Nursing Administration*[1]

BY DOREEN WEDDELL

Human relations in administration is an odd phrase, for what is administration but a system of relationships, formal and informal, between a number of people, which enables a process to occur, makes it possible for things to be done conveniently and speedily? Theoretically, relationships will be satisfactory if the right person for the job has been chosen (and methods of selection come in here), if it is clear to whom and for what she is responsible, and if there are adequate opportunities for everyone to meet to discuss planning and the difficulties that arise in the course of the work. By and large, most people can get on with most other people unless one or other of them is ill in himself.

In practice, however, it is not always easy to find the right person for the job. The position of ward sister seems to require someone who not only is a skilful bedside nurse, but can experience within herself the disturbance of the patient and relatives and upsets of the staff, yet keep outside the upheaval so that she may seek ways of dealing with the situation clearly and calmly.

It may not be difficult to define the task of the ward sister, as expert nurse, as nurse teacher, as ward administrator, but it is not always clear to whom she is responsible.

WARD RELATIONSHIPS

Let us look at the structure of ward administration as it is in many hospitals today, that is, the system of relationships between the ward sister and various members of the staff and others who go to

[1] Reprinted from a paper given at a ward sisters' conference, Royal College of Nursing, and published in the *Nursing Times*, 30 December 1955.

the ward. What is her role in relation to each of these? For what is she really responsible? For what does she *feel* responsible, though she may not have the authority that makes it possible for her to do anything about it?

In the first place, who is really responsible for the patient? He is said to be the focus of our attention, the centre of our interest, but who is ultimately responsible for him? If you ask the patient, he may say the sister, the nurse, or the doctor; if you ask the nurse, she may say the sister or the doctor– and some matrons may consider that they are responsible. Poor patient! When should he be allowed to be responsible for himself and by whom? The hospital provides a service for his benefit, but should he be allowed to choose how he will use it, or be taken control of from the moment of admission, told what to do, when to do it, what is good for him, bad for him, and by whom? How far should he really be allowed to know what is happening to him, so that he can make a reasoned choice about his future? None of us is as clear about these matters as we should like to be.

If we are not always clear about who is responsible for the patient, what about the ward sister? To whom is she responsible? From whom does she in practice take her orders, and for what has she actual authority? It is worth pointing out here that a sound principle of administration is that no one should be responsible to more than one person. If there are conflicting allegiances or interests, there will be anxiety, tension, and even breakdown.[1] This is true for patients and staff.

It is not enough – though it is a lot – to get the right person for the job, a reasonably able person, with adequate skill and interest in people, and to give her all the equipment and staff she requires for her work. We need to plan also the system of relationships that she may have to sustain in her day-to-day work. *Figure 1* shows the number of relationships the ward sister may have in any one day in a ward where group or case assignment is not the method of nursing. There may be four or five doctors coming to the ward – the ward sister wants to see each of them; there are six or seven nursing staff, also a physiotherapist, an occupational therapist, a social worker, a dietitian, a laboratory technician, and theatre staff; there are the matron, the deputy matron, the tutor, and administrative personnel; as well as twenty-five or so patients and their relatives.

[1] See also Chapter 26 – Ed.

In other words, by all the rules, the ward sister is in an impossible position, pulled this way and that by conflicting requirements, by the needs of people whose priority is not clearly defined. She feels she has to do one thing to please the doctor, something else because the matron's office wants it, the theatre sister wants

FIGURE I Ward sister's relationships

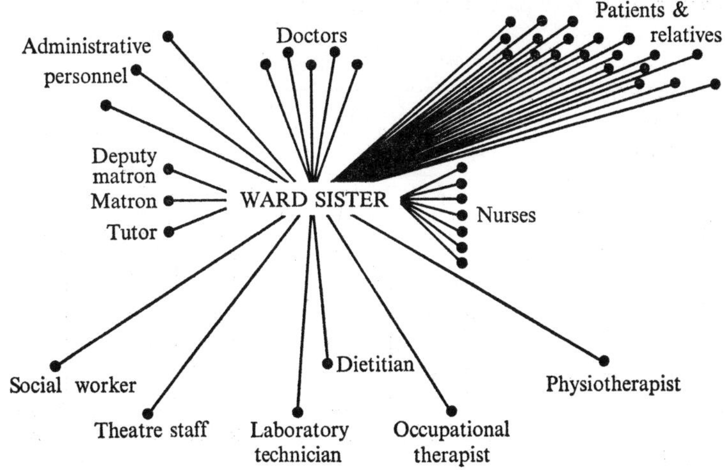

something different, the tutor says something else, and relatives want her attention at the same moment. How can she deal with so many demands?

Some people manage by extreme orderliness, an absolutely rigid timetable and no relaxation for special requests. This seems to work quite well, but it may be rather like sitting on a volcano, which will erupt with chaos if any controls are loosened. Other people expend themselves in an endless attempt to meet all the demands. Some people just give up hope and abdicate from the situation. Most ward sisters struggle along, vaguely feeling that somebody should do something, not very sure what it should be, and at different times thinking it is the doctor, the matron, or the administrative staff who should lighten their task.

One way of improving relationships in the ward seems to be through delegation of work, giving absolute responsibility and adequate authority to the people to whom it is delegated, so that everything does not have to be channelled through the ward sister. Case assignment, small group assignment, team care of patients, are ways of accomplishing this, with the advantage to the patient that he is able to know precisely where he comes in the picture, that he is someone's particular concern. Similarly, the nurse can have the satisfaction of devoting her energies to a few people instead of having to divide her interest among all the patients in the ward.

FIGURE 2 A new pattern of relationships

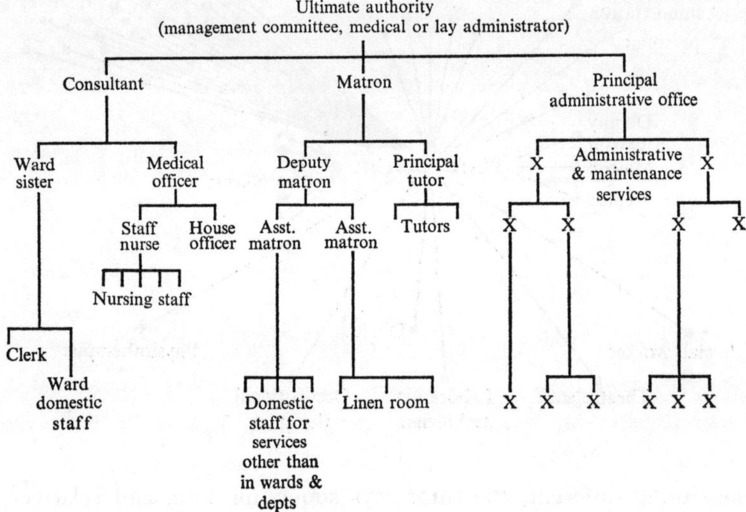

To many ward sisters such a suggestion is felt as an undermining of their authority, a taking away of what they most enjoy in their work. They feel that they must know everything that is going on in the ward or something is sure to go wrong. There is, however, a difference between *knowing* what is going on, that is, having adequate channels of communication, and *feeling responsible* for everything that happens. Some ward sisters will say that young people today do not like responsibility. What will the ward sister have to do, where will her satisfaction come from, if she delegates so much of her work? Before answering these questions, let us look at *Figure 2*.[1]

[1] Readers are reminded that this paper was written in 1955, some years before the appointment of domestic supervisors became common practice in hospitals and eleven years before the publication of the Salmon Report on Senior Nursing Staff Structure (Ministry of Health, 1966).

Figure 2 shows what an administrative structure defining working relationships could look like, when responsibility is to one person only and when authority and responsibility are delegated. It is a hypothetical diagram but illustrates the possible relationships between a ward (where group assignment of patients is in operation), the matron's office, and the administrative office. Up and down are the formal executive relationships; crosswise are the informal relationships, whereby one section may *request* services from the other.

If the ward unit is taken as the basic one, then all other departments can be regarded as providing services for that unit. The matron can be said to recruit and allocate the trained nursing staff for the ward unit; she provides a service of training for unskilled staff and delegates the task of training nurses to the tutors, who, in turn, will allocate the students to the ward sister for training purposes. The ward sister will then allocate nursing staff to doctors and thus to patients. The diagram shows the staff nurse as responsible to the medical officer and that there are nurses responsible to her. For a large ward this grouping would be repeated. A ward arranged in a different way might show the staff nurse responsible to the sister.

Figure 2 illustrates that it is possible to have a system of relationships very different from that shown in *Figure 1*. The important point is that each ward, each department, each hospital, needs a definition of roles and relationships which can be portrayed. When a ward sister starts trying to define the structure in her particular ward and hospital, she will no doubt find that there are many other questions to settle. For instance, to whom should the night nurse be responsible? To the night sister? Or should she be a member of the ward team, responsible to the house doctor?

In industry and in newspaper offices, these things are very clearly defined and it is considered essential for heads of departments and sections to meet regularly if the job is to be efficiently completed on time. Often these concerns, like the hospital, have to provide a round-the-clock service, though their work may not be quite so much a matter of life and death. In the hospital world, not enough time would seem to be spent on getting together within departments or by departments. How many ward sisters have called a conference of all those who come to the ward to discuss such a matter as noise? How many would know what channels of communication to use for this purpose?

WARD SISTER'S ROLE[1]

Let us now return to the question of the ward sister's role, and the work she could do and the satisfaction she might get if she delegated many of her present-day tasks.

She can be the *provider of services* for staff and patients; the *personnel officer* for the staff of the ward and the patients' relatives; the *presenter* – she can present the ward's interests and needs to other departments, she can present the interests and needs of one section of the staff to another, those of patients and relatives to each other, to the hospital authorities, and so on. Under this last heading come all her teaching activities. She presents a point of view, a way of doing things.

As provider of ward services, the ward sister will be an expert in getting what she wants for the ward. More than that, she will get what the staff and patients feel they want. That is, she not only thinks on their behalf, but encourages them to think out and express their needs, so that what is obtained is really what is wanted.

At the Cassel Hospital, a certain amount of money is allocated yearly to each ward (or unit, as they are called) for repairs and renewals of furniture, furnishing, crockery, equipment, and redecoration. Each ward budgets how it will spend the money. The plan is formulated by the ward sister as the customer, in consultation with the rest of the staff and the patients. It is the supplies officer's task to see that she gets what she wants within her budget. Such a procedure may not be possible in every hospital, but it is surprising what can be done, and nurses enjoy being housewife for the ward in this way.

As personnel officer, the ward sister can become as interested and as expert in diagnosing and treating the upsets of relationships that occur in the ward as she has hitherto been in the nursing treatment of the patient.

Stanton and Schwartz (1954) have shown that unexpressed disagreement between staff affects patients' behaviour. Their work was done with psychiatric patients, but if a similar situation was inves-

[1] See also Chapter 26 – Ed.

tigated in a general hospital, much the same sort of thing might be found. We need to know much more about the occasions when the nurse has not really agreed with something that the doctor has ordered, the thing has gone wrong, and she has secretly said to herself, 'I told you so'. The ward sister as personnel officer to the ward can do something to sort out such situations. She will be concerned with the relationships of the ward staff and all who visit the ward; porters, technicians, medical auxiliaries, relatives, will all be seen as an essential part of the ward team. If the visitors' relationship with the ward personnel is satisfactory then the patient is likely to receive the best possible benefit from their visit.

At present, the ward sister is the one most concerned with relatives and patients' visitors, their interests and anxieties; but eventually the nurse actually looking after the patient might be the one to whom the relatives will turn. As the nurse in training comes to feel the patient not as her property, but as a member of his own family,[1] she will also see as part of her nursing task the understanding, maintaining, and fostering of patients' family ties during the interruption of illness, and will become skilled in this function.

In other words, though in delegating much of her present-day work the ward sister may feel she is losing all that really interests her, in fact she may be able to find new satisfactions and new skills, and come to feel as proud of the way in which the staff of the ward 'grow up' and achieve things as she was of the patients she actually nursed.

THE MATRON'S OFFICE

The matron's office can set the pattern for this way of viewing the human relationships of administration. How the matron works with the ward sisters may be reflected in how they work with their staff nurses, and they in turn with student nurses. The matron's office can be thought of as a kind of 'grandmotherly home' – a place where ward sisters go to talk about their problems, their ideas and aspirations, their anxieties about staff, about patients and relatives, a place where there is time to be heard and to listen. An hour a week or a fortnight, or even once a month – an hour the ward sister can use as she wishes, to grumble about something, to

[1] See also Chapter 21 – Ed.

obtain information, to ask advice. This is the conception of the matron as personnel officer to her staff. It means that she must be clear, and so must the sisters, about her role and what relationship may be needed at any one time – that of employer, adviser, teacher, or confidante.

Administration or personnel work, however, does not just mean running around keeping everybody happy. The task is to see that the work goes smoothly and if there is a difficulty to see what it is about and to seek ways of solving it to the satisfaction of all concerned, including oneself. How can this be done? In the Cassel Hospital it is easy to meet patients informally, so a ward round as such is not done very often, but a visit is paid by the matron to each ward sister's office every morning[1] to hear from her the events of the day, any problems there may be, who is being awkward with whom, how a particularly ill patient may be affecting the staff and other patients, and so on. The ward sister may ask the nurse who is looking after the particularly ill patient[2] to come and talk about what is happening, or there may be a discussion concerning a patient's convalescence or a family situation that is difficult. Often it is not necessary to say very much; the opportunity to put the problem into words may be enough to set the staff thinking of new ways of solving it. Sometimes asking the question 'Whose problem is this really?' will put the whole matter into perspective and allow the nurse to see how over-concerned she may be getting about something that she can affect only to a very small extent. In any event, what is said is only in the form of *advice*. From her experience, the matron can put as broad a point of view as possible before the ward sister so that the latter can make her own choice in the light of all the information she can get.

Administrative procedures relating to off-duty have, in the past, often caused tension between the matron's office and the ward. Who should decide this? If nurses are allocated to a ward, is their off-duty any longer the concern of the matron except in general principle? Should the ward sister decide it, or can it be delegated to the team? Is the ward sister free to make such arrangements as best suit her ward? Can each team be a law to itself or should two teams cover each other? If it is decided to delegate this task, it is

[1] This arrangement was in operation at the time of writing – Ed.

[2] Case assignment, whereby one nurse looks after six to ten patients, has been in operation at the Cassel Hospital since 1946 – Ed.

possible also to set the framework within which the team has freedom to operate; for instance, that there must always be a nurse in the ward, that certain procedures must be accomplished between certain hours. If the ward sister is wise, she will have discussed and got agreement even on this framework before delegating the task. If the team has to work out for itself how to cover the ward, taking into account that some people have to go to lectures, some have boy friends and want evenings off, others have evening classes on a particular night, others like to go shopping in the mornings, the end-result is much more likely to be satisfactory to all concerned than if one person decides it.

It is important to be clear about when we really are *delegating* a job and when we are *consulting* with our staff. In consultation we ask our staff for advice, we discuss their needs, or we may ask them to tell us what they want and say that we will agree to it. We may say, 'I want to know what you want. I may not be able to agree, but I'll do the best I can.' The final decision is ours. Once we have delegated the task, however, advice may be sought from us on how it might be carried out, or we may offer suggestions, but the choice, the decision about the matter, will be made by the person to whom the task is delegated.

WARD SISTER AND TUTOR

A brief indication of the ward sister's role as the presenter has been given, but one other point about her role in teaching and her relationship with the tutor might be made.

If the tutor is responsible for training the student nurse, then for some portion of her time the ward sister (and the staff nurse) could be considered responsible to the tutor. In this case the sister would have two relationships with the tutor. As personnel officer she would advise the tutor on how the student was progressing in her ward work and relationships, emotionally, intellectually, and physically. The tutor would, however, be able to instruct the ward sister about what things she should teach the student in the ward.

There are other ways of looking at and dealing with this question, as with others already mentioned. Each has distinct merits. What is important, however, is that the relationship of tutor, ward sister, and student nurse should be clearly defined so that each knows where she is and where the others are, when to instruct and give advice, when obedience is necessary, when there is a choice of conduct, when a service is being provided which may be accepted or rejected.

THE CHILD IN THE ADULT

Why are these practical aspects of administration so important? Why this emphasis on knowing roles and responsibility, on channels of communication, on formal and informal relationships, delegation of authority, and methods of consultation?

When we think back to childhood, and there is something of the child in all of us, occasions will be recalled when we felt hurt, resentful, angry, because something was going on and we were not allowed to know much about it, not allowed in; or we were made to do things, go to places, and we did not understand what was going on – at such moments it is natural to hate everyone around us, and to be jealous of brothers and sisters old enough to be in the know. The essence of administration is to explain what is going on and why, to listen, watch, assess the effect; to give a feeling of belonging, of being valued, seeking to obviate childish responses in patients, staff, and relatives.

At one time or another most children have felt that they could get more out of father than mother, and vice versa, or that if anything was wanted mother had to be got round first, or perhaps father. Most children have told tales on brothers or sisters, either to get the other child into trouble or for some momentary gain. Some adults tend to go on doing this sort of thing, though not always very obviously or directly; others hated being told what to do when they were children, and still feel rebellious when in a similar position as adults.

Some of us, as children, were more suspicious than others of what was being plotted against us, of what things were being taken away from us or which of us was first in mother's or father's affections. Jealousy and envy of older or younger brothers' and sisters' possessions and position are frequent in children, and can be seen later in adults' problems of status, promotion, and so on. Providing a clearly defined administrative structure, which allows everyone to know where he stands in relation to everyone else, can be said to be like providing a stable home background. In a secure home, a child can know where he stands with his parents and his brothers and sisters, when he can be adventurous, when he can use his initiative, when he must conform and obey; his guile, avarice, and capacity to set one person against the other can be seen for what they are with the minimum of disturbance to the family. So the administrative structure can give security, can make for freedom, yet within known limits. A bad administrative structure confuses and frustrates staff. But a sound administrative structure is not *by itself* enough. Satisfactory relationships for all concerned will depend on how the structure is used, whether in an authoritarian manner, or with consultation, and this in turn will depend on the characteristics of the people who fill the roles that comprise the focal points in the structure.

It is when roles become equated with status that there is likely to be trouble. Some people carry responsibility easily, other people's anxieties about this may result in a need to keep everything very much under control, and their attention to detail may mean that human matters are lost sight of. It may be difficult for such people to accept advice or suggestions because these are felt as attacks upon their position. One reason for this may be that inside themselves they feel they have to be the perfect parent who should know everything and always have the right answer, the kind of parent they wanted when they were children. The attacks, taunts, demands they made as children are now re-experienced as coming from the people with whom they work. Just as some parents are so anxious lest their child should come to harm in some way that they hedge him round with dos and don'ts and protect him from every potentially dangerous situation, so in administration such people make it difficult for anyone with whom they are working to try out, test, and experience the capacities within themselves.

It is well for a ward sister to remember that she cannot help but be, to some extent, a parent substitute to the staff and patients of the ward. She may be made out to be a monster, or be over-idealized, depending on how these particular patients and staff have mainly felt about their parents and people in authority from infancy until the present day. Some people need to be able to put the blame on to someone or something outside themselves. This is not only something that individuals do but a process that may occur in any group or community. Some one person or department may be felt to be the focus of irritation, the cause of all the trouble, that all would be well if only someone or something were different.

Though the ward sister or staff nurse may frequently fill this role for the ward group, it sometimes happens that a student nurse becomes the scapegoat.

Where the ward sister is idealized there will be an increased need to see someone else as bad and awkward, to be the repository of the aggressive, destructive feelings that must not be directed towards her, and the tutor may sometimes seem to come in at this point. In turn, the ward sister will see and feel for the various members of the staff and the patients of the ward in a way that is characteristically hers. They may be predominantly children to be cared for or protected, rivals to be fought with or controlled, or individuals with rights, experiences, and wishes of their own, with whom it is possible to have an easy reciprocal relationship in which each can give to and take from the other.

Where these various pictures and needs are roughly commensurate, relationships will be reasonably good, and a defined structure will assist the process; but where there is gross distortion there will be trouble, however good the administrative structure may be. Defining the administrative structure, the roles and responsibilities in an organization, will not of itself improve or solve difficulties of human relationships, but it will make it easier to see what is happening.

It is not possible to conclude without making some reference to the question of achieving change. Much will depend on the quality of the relationships in the framework within which change is sought – for even a minor modification of procedures necessitates some change of feeling and thinking within the individuals concerned. Acceptance of change is more likely to occur when the proposed change can be thoroughly discussed by all concerned, with decisions and methods of implementation agreed before any alteration is introduced. There are sometimes, however, very strong unrecognizable motives for collusion, for maintaining the *status quo*, and then advice or help from someone outside the situation is necessary.

26 · *The Role of the Ward Sister*[1]

BY EILEEN SKELLERN

The following is the report of an investigation, the terms of reference of which were, 'to study, report and make recommendations on the practical application to ward administration of modern methods in the instruction and handling of staff and student nurses'.

In the author's view a ward is a living, moving 'organism' with an internal organization central to the carrying out of certain objectives. Although it is within a geographical location of four walls in a hospital building, which gives it an apparent isolation, it is, in fact, dependent for its existence upon the hospital, as the hospital, in turn, is upon the community. Looked at in this way, each ward, like a living organism, has unique characteristics of its own as well as many in common with other organisms of the same species. Wards do not differ so much in the tasks they carry out or in the techniques they develop to organize these tasks. These are usually easy to describe. They vary much more, however, with regard to their complicated systems of internal and external, formal and informal relationships, for these are intangible and constantly

[1] This chapter is reprinted from a monograph published by the Royal College of Nursing in 1953. The investigation was initiated by the Ward and Departmental Sisters' Section of the Royal College of Nursing, and financed by a bursary awarded by Messrs Boots the Chemists.

Many people assisted the author. She wishes particularly to mention Isobel E. P. Menzies, of the Tavistock Institute of Human Relations, for her valuable contribution to the organization and execution of the project. The author, being a nurse, and a ward sister at the time, found it easier to identify and understand the problems of certain sections of the hospital staff than others. Miss Menzies helped to prevent too great a degree of subjectivity, to maintain a continuous review of the field method and research design in relation to the data as they came in, and to analyse the data in terms of sociological and psychological concepts.

changing. In this sense, each ward is unique. Description of any one ward is difficult and it is impossible to find and portray an average ward. The report, therefore, seeks to examine certain principles governing the life of the ward, with examples taken from observation of fifty-seven wards.

PLAN OF WORK

The aim was to study ward problems of administration, training, and relationships, and some of the methods used to solve these problems. The plan was to proceed through a series of steps, from an extensive and fairly superficial survey of hospital life in general, which would indicate some of the general characteristics of wards, to a more detailed study of one hospital, which would yield fuller information about the relationship of ward to hospital, and, finally, to an even more intensive study of a single ward. In this way, it was felt that deeper insight and more intimate knowledge would be gained concerning the workings of the ward and its internal and external relationships.

FIELDWORK

The hospital field

(*a*) Background material was gained by:

consulting specialists in nursing, administration, and training at the Royal College of Nursing, the Ministry of Health, the Ministry of Labour, and the King's Fund College of Hospital Management;

meeting groups of matrons, tutors, ward and departmental sisters, other trained nurses and student nurses through the Royal College of Nursing;

visiting an independent school of nursing run on group lines in the north of England;

attending conferences at the Royal College of Nursing;

visiting the team undertaking a hospital job analysis sponsored by the Nuffield Provincial Hospital Trust;

studying a research project undertaken by Miss M. J. Johnson, B.Sc., Ph.D. (Birmingham), of University College, London, concerned with the use of group methods in the selection and training of medical students;

reading relevant literature and the nursing periodicals, the *Nursing Times* and the *Nursing Mirror*.

(b) Selection of the hospitals to be visited was to some extent influenced by the advice of the Ward Sisters' Section of the Royal College of Nursing. The aim was first to visit a representative cross-section of general and specialized teaching and non-teaching hospitals in the United Kingdom. At the same time, wherever possible, more than one hospital in a city was visited in order to take in a cross-section of the hospitals in one place (see *Table 2*). The length of time spent in a hospital varied from half a day to three days.

In order to gain understanding of the relationship of the ward to the hospital as a whole, one week was spent in a teaching hospital of 833 beds in the north of England. The three main departmental groupings – medical, nursing, and administrative – were visited. Staff at many levels were interviewed: for example, consultants, registrars, housemen, and medical students in the medical group; the matron and her deputies, tutors, home sisters, departmental and ward sisters, staff nurses and student nurses in the nursing group; and heads of departments, supervisors, clerks, secretaries, kitchen staff, porters, and cleaners in the third group.

A medical ward of twenty-eight beds in a London teaching hospital of 697 beds was selected for the intensive study. Daily observations of a few hours' duration were made over a period of three weeks, and the times were planned so that the twenty-four-hour cycle was covered during the three weeks. The three main spheres of interest were the ward team, the patients, and staff visiting the ward. The three main functions of the nursing staff, nursing, administration, and teaching (or being trained), were considered, and the matron, her deputy, night sisters, and tutors were interviewed.

The Industrial Field

It had been planned initially to obtain comparative material from the industrial sphere. Time, however, did not allow either an extensive study of the industrial field or an intensive study of

TABLE 2 HOSPITALS VISITED

Area	*Number of beds*	*Type of hospital*	*Teaching or non-teaching*
London	60	Psychiatric	Non-teaching
	104	Psychiatric	Non-teaching
	239	General	Teaching
	337	General	Non-teaching
	400	General	Non-teaching
	408	General	Non-teaching
	409	General	Teaching
	491	General	Teaching
	519	General	Teaching
	544	General	Teaching
	562	Orthopaedic	Teaching
	697	General	Teaching
South-West England	697	General	Teaching
Midlands	657	General	Non-teaching
	373	General	Teaching
North-West England 1 City	136	Children's	Non-teaching
	661	Children's	Teaching
	816	General	Non-teaching
North-East England	833	General	Teaching
Wales 1 City	368	General	Teaching
	328	General	Non-teaching
	219	Fever	—
Scotland 1 City	625	General	Teaching
	1,588	General	Non-teaching
	503	General	Non-teaching
	55	Convalescent	—

problems of relationships within industry. Priority was given, therefore, to the hospital field and its problems. It was possible, nevertheless, to consider superficially certain aspects of industrial management and training, and the techniques devised by some of the more progressive factories to meet their problems. Four factories were visited – one of them a number of times (*Table 3*).

TABLE 3 FACTORIES VISITED

Area	*Type of manufacture*
South-West England	Tobacco and cigarettes
South-East England	Radio and plastics
London	Cars
	Metal ball bearings

Background material was obtained by consulting specialists in administration, consultation, and training at the Ministry of Labour, the Tavistock Institute of Human Relations, and the Social Science Department of Liverpool University, and by reading relevant literature.

ELICITING AND EVALUATING DATA

Interviewing

(*a*) Individual people were interviewed while at their work. The open method of interviewing was used rather than the questionnaire, as being more suitable for the eliciting of material concerning relationships. Each interview began with a brief account of the investigation, followed by an invitation to the interviewee to talk about her own work in her own way. From that point, the interviewee set the pace and course of the interview, which lasted from a quarter of an hour to one hour according to the time available. Notes were not taken at the time but were written up as soon as possible afterwards.

(*b*) A number of groups of people were interviewed, varying in size from eight to thirty people. The technique employed was similar to that used when interviewing individuals. The investigator spoke of the investigation and then allowed the group to develop free discussion on its own lines. Where the group was composed of a cross-section of the hospital staff, for example, matrons, tutors, sisters, and so on, it re-created some of the interpersonal relationships commonly seen in the hospital, each person drawing from her own experience. This helped the investigator to evaluate the situation, and at the same time allowed the group to examine many facets of any one problem. When the group was composed entirely of one type of staff, for example ward sisters or student nurses, the common problems of that group were more clearly seen. Whatever the composition of the group, the results were invaluable in enlarging the background material of the investigation.

Observation

Wherever possible the investigator wore a white coat, rather than a nurse's uniform, to minimize identification with any one section of the ward team. Observations were then made in the course of active participation in aspects of ward work so that the investigation was carried on under as near to normal working conditions as possible and the ward routine was not impeded.

OBJECTIVES OF THE HOSPITAL

The three main objectives of the hospital are:

to treat the patient;
to train staff to do this;
to carry out research.

The organization of the hospital evolved to achieve these aims.

TREATMENT

The patient comes to the hospital complaining of certain symptoms and asking to be cured. The hospital is concerned in the care of the patient, investigating his diagnosis and prescribing and carrying out the treatment of his disease. The patient's disease usually follows a certain pattern whatever its origin: from the onset, through the acute phase, to convalescence and partial or complete recovery, or to relapse and death. The pattern is conditioned by the degree of illness and examples of all stages can be seen in the hospital ward.

Treatment, however, implies more than treatment of a specific disease. The physical and psychological aspects cannot be considered separately for, whether the disease be primarily physical or psychological in origin, the person as a whole will be affected. The patient is a member of a family, with work, interests, and ties outside the hospital. The illness and its treatment are of great importance to himself and his family, however slight the illness may be. In order to receive treatment the patient is asked for the time being to relinquish these outward ties either partially or completely; to give up his independence, along with his clothes, and become a passive, dependent person. If he is acutely ill this dependency may be welcomed, but if he walks into the hospital, as so many patients do, he may feel resentful and want to retain his adult status.

During treatment the patient has to face not only bodily discomfort and pain but emotional and mental strain. He will react according to the stage of his illness, being very dependent if acutely ill or possibly fractious and difficult when recovering. He will have anxiety and worries about his home situation, his expectations of treatment, and his chances of recovery. Such anxieties are intensified by deep fears which are frequently unexpressed or unformulated even in his own mind. In addition, he has to cope with separation from home and adapt to a new mode of life with its own peculiar rules, living with people who are suffering, and perhaps seeing death for the first time. All these factors impress him and may have a direct effect on the rate of his recovery.

Treatment, therefore, is a wide term used to cover the diagnosis and treatment of the patient's specific disease and the care of the patient with both physical and psychological needs. To treat the patient, the hospital asks him to adopt a dependent role and at the same time sanctions the staff to be active on his behalf.

TRAINING

All staff, irrespective of the type of work they do, have to learn how to carry out their work. The length of training varies according to the skill and knowledge required so that doctors and nurses have a longer training than, for example, domestic staff. The training of the student nurse aims at teaching her to carry out the instructions of the doctor, and to understand and deal with people both in sickness and in health. In the same way that the patient cannot be considered divorced from society, so, too, the nurse belongs to the same society and her training should prepare her to accept the responsibilities of her position in that society.

The nurse needs to have sufficient theoretical knowledge of the normal and abnormal physical and psychological make-up of the individual to enable her to understand and carry out the doctors' instructions intelligently and safely. Her training teaches her the techniques of nursing procedure for the specific and general care of the patient and how to prepare and maintain equipment necessary to carry out this procedure. She has to learn how to apply the nursing procedure to the patient as an individual and to understand and reassure him in difficulty whenever possible. The nurse learns to observe and report on the patient's condition and the effects of her ministrations and to act promptly and wisely in times of emergency. She learns how to work with others and take responsibility, and how to administer and care for equipment and the hospital building as well as the patient.

The nurse, therefore, needs to be trained to fill a role with many facets: to nurse; to teach staff, patients, and their relatives positive and preventive health; to administer; and to take her place as a responsible citizen in society. Systems of training vary, but, on the whole, theory and the technique of practical nursing are taught by the tutor in the classroom, using a study day or block system for the purpose. Practical nursing is carried out in the wards and the nurse is moved every two or three months to give her as varied experience in technical nursing as possible over a span of three years.

RESEARCH

This is a term commonly applied in hospital only to scientific experiments in the diagnosis of disease and the discovery of new drugs and techniques of treatment. But if research is to be considered in its widest sense, then all grades and kinds of staff have an essential contribution to make to further the advance of medical and other knowledge for the benefit of present and future patients. For example, observations of patients' condition and behaviour, the perfection of nursing technique, examination of and experimentation in ward and hospital administration, and methods of teaching, may be the contribution of the nursing staff to the total picture.

SOME PROBLEMS OF FULFILMENT

It is difficult to achieve a balance in the attainment of these objectives at one and the same time and, inevitably, sacrifice in the common interest must be made by first one group then another.

It would appear that clinical interest in the patient's disease frequently causes the staff to forget the patient as a person with individual rights and feelings. For example, a clinical teaching session was given on a woman aged thirty-five, the mother of a large family. She heard indirectly, for the first time, through remarks addressed to the students who were present, that her heart condition would necessitate drastic restriction in her activities when she left hospital. This left no possibility of dealing effectively with the emotional upset which such information inevitably caused.

The clinical interest of the disease may so absorb the staff that they forget that the patient can see, hear, and use his intelligence even though ill in bed. Too often ward rounds are made without the patient saying or contributing anything himself though he is talked about in his hearing. Often he may be kept in ignorance of his disease and progress, even on discharge from hospital. During the course of this investigation it was enlightening to note that many patients in the ward did, in fact, find out their own and other people's diagnosis and prognosis through watching, overhearing remarks, and asking questions, especially of medical and nursing students. The picture they were able to build from these scraps of information was frequently distorted and inaccurate, raising rather than alleviating anxiety and fear. This state of affairs is due not so much to negligence on the part of the staff as to lack of appreciation of the patient's point of view, of the kind of emotional disturbance that their attitude engenders, and its effect on the patient's recovery.

The conflicting claims on student nurses for staffing and training were evident. Instead of being given work to do which aimed at supplementing their training, the pressure of work and shortage of staff in so many hospitals made it difficult for them to be considered primarily as students.

HISTORICAL DEVELOPMENT OF THE HOSPITAL SYSTEM

THE HOSPITAL IN SOCIETY

The problem of the sick person in society has been tackled in a variety of ways according to the age. During the Middle Ages two forms of hospital existed, those provided by the monasteries as part of their pastoral duties and those provided by the Crusaders to house the wounded.

After the reformation and the dissolution of the monasteries, the majority of infirmaries and hospitals fell into disuse. The burden of the care of the sick and poor was taken over by the villages and towns, but this system proved inadequate when the large-scale migration from country to town began in the early nineteenth century at the start of the industrial revolution. At this time, conditions in the factories, sweated labour, child labour, and crowded living conditions contributed to an increase in disease and a high mortality rate. The time was ripe for social reform of all kinds. Many new hospitals were built and existing ones were changed from being dirty, infection-ridden, feared institutions into comparatively clean, smooth-running places, largely owing to the influence of Florence Nightingale in the second half of the nineteenth century.

As medical and nursing knowledge expanded, more hospitals were founded, especially in the late nineteenth and early twentieth centuries. They were governed, financed, and administered by a variety of bodies. One group became the voluntary hospital system, another the municipal hospital system, and there were many small private hospitals. This irregular development continued until 1948 when the national health service combined all hospitals in one service controlled by the state through parliament, with the exception of certain privately owned nursing homes.

MEDICAL RESEARCH AND TREATMENT

It is impossible to do more than indicate milestones in the development of medical knowledge and treatment. Originally, disease was thought to be caused by evil spirits, and superstitions still govern some people's attitude to illness. Scientific development in this country started in the seventeenth century when normal and abnormal anatomy and physiology were studied. Later, Pasteur and other scientists were able to isolate bacteriological causes of disease and show how infectious diseases were spread.

At first diagnosis depended on the history of symptoms and observable and palpable signs on examination. X-rays and modern pathology have created a speciality of diagnosis. Treatment advanced rapidly after the introduction of anaesthetics, surgical techniques were made safer by antiseptic and aseptic precautions, knowledge of drugs and chemotherapy increased.

Social medicine with its keynote of prevention has contributed greatly to the prevention of disease by better housing and sanitation, food laws, vaccination, immunization, maternity welfare, and school care. The result of all this is longer expectation of life which, in turn, gives rise to the current pressing problems concerning the ageing sick and geriatric care.

Psychiatric knowledge, in particular psycho-analysis, has contributed not only to the diagnosis and treatment of mental disorders but to the understanding of human behaviour and its development, influencing education, the care of children, and attitudes to crime. Psychosomatic medicine gives evidence of the close relationship between physical and psychological illness so that increasing attention is paid to the patient as a whole person, giving rise to a new era of psychosocial medicine.

PERSONNEL

The rapid growth of medical knowledge created the need for all kinds of staff in many fields of health work. In the past, the care of the patient has been undertaken by first one group of people then another. In the Middle Ages, the monks and nuns cared for the whole patient, concentrating on food, shelter, spiritual comfort, and palliative remedies to ease pain, rather than on investigating the cause of the disease. After the dissolution of the monasteries, the barber-surgeons were interested in the disease but not in the nursing and care of the patient. With the exception of certain holy orders who continued their ministrations throughout, care of the patient was left to anyone – servants or relatives at home and drunks and ne'er-do-wells in hospital.

When Florence Nightingale revolutionized nursing in the last century, replacing the dissipated uneducated women with educated, hardworking, self-sacrificing nurses, she laid the foundation of the present hospital nursing service. For the first time, two groups of people worked side by side in the hospital, the doctors and the nurses. The nurses proved so capable that more was delegated to them, leaving the doctor to concentrate on the patient's disease itself while the nurse administered, cleaned the ward, and nursed the patient.

As treatment, skill, and knowledge became more specialized, more staff were introduced. The nursing staff were relieved of some cleaning by domestic staff, of food preparation by dietitians, and of social work by almoners. The doctors delegated diagnosis and special therapeutic treatments to pathologists, bacteriologists, physiotherapists, and so on. Gradually a complex hospital service has developed, each part giving specialized knowledge and skill to the care and treatment of the patient.

SOME PROBLEMS OF SPECIALIZATION

Specialization in a certain aspect of the patient's disease tends to make the specialist concentrate on the part at the expense of the whole of the patient. As medical knowledge advances, the need to see the patient as a whole entity becomes apparent, highlighting the necessity for co-ordination of the team in the interests both of treatment and of the patient as an individual.

A patient when very ill is dependent on those who care for him. Thus a unique relationship is created between the patient and those who come into contact with him, especially the nurse. A very sick patient is like a child in that he has the child's limited capacity for making relationships and can cope only with one or two people. Any additional strain combined with his illness tires the patient. For the patient who is not so ill the strain is less but may still be bewildering. The relationship between nurse and patient is not dissimilar to that seen in the family between the mother and the small child. Like the mother, the nurse may become protective and possessive of the patient. This may be good for the patient who is very ill and in need of security, provided it is given up at the appropriate point. At the same time, the number of people authorized to question and examine the patient has increased. He must talk to and make relationships with many more people. A close relationship develops between patient, nurse, and doctor. This, combined with the irregular historical development of staff functions, may subsequently contribute to tension between specialist groups. The basic group of patient, doctor, and nurse may feel the others to be intruders.

Newer treatments mean more rapid recovery. This directly affects the nurse and a ward organization which was based on the patients' slower recovery rate. Early ambulation and shortened stay in hospital have altered the art and satisfactions of nursing, making speed and pressure greater. For example, the patient suffering from pneumonia largely depended in the past on the skill of the nurse to bring him through the crisis; this created a special bond between the two. Today, chemotherapy minimizes the dangers of many such diseases, curing more patients but curtailing some of the nursing satisfactions. Nursing skills have to be adapted to meet new demands.

BASIC ORGANIZATION OF HOSPITAL AND WARD

Ward organization has to be seen in relation to the hospital as a whole, and hospital structure has to be considered in relation to the national health service.

THE NATIONAL HEALTH SERVICE

The Ministry of Health frames its overall policy on the needs of the service and the available resources in money and manpower. The Minister is responsible to the country through parliament for providing a national health service. In the curative field, this responsibility is divided between two main groups, the hospital service and the domiciliary service. The hospital service is the responsibility of regional hospital boards and boards of governors. The regional hospital boards, in turn, delegate their responsibility to hospital management committees who, in turn, provide a service for the general practitioner and are provided with certain services from the domiciliary side for the benefit of the patient.

The National Health Service Act of 1946 clearly defines who is responsible for the patient. This falls to the doctor, the one clinical staff member to be appointed direct by the regional hospital board. The Minister provides the building and the hospital management committee the services for the use of the doctor. The services are medical auxiliary, nursing, domestic, and administrative. The head of each service is responsible to the hospital management committee for providing that service and for its administration.

HOSPITAL STRUCTURE

The framework of the hospital is based on a system of interrelated hierarchies, a structure whereby a system of interdependent roles is created, each responsible to and for another. The senior person in each hierarchy is responsible for the whole hierarchy and delegates this responsibility accordingly down the line of control. There are three main hierarchical groups in the hospital: medical, nursing, and administrative. Each hierarchy has a number of functions. Each provides a system of promotion, a structure for the administration of a service, and the supply of staff to working units.

FIGURE 3 A system of promotion

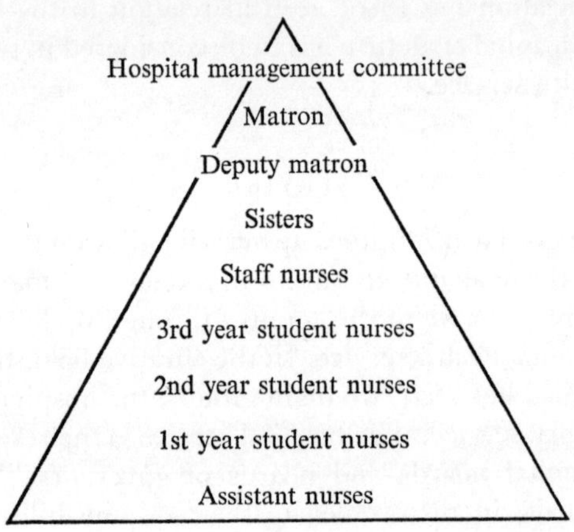

Figure 3 illustrates a system of promotion. The nursing group as a whole is graded in a hierarchy in this manner, which does not necessarily imply responsibility to the person directly above or for the person directly below. Promotion is achieved by passing from one grade to another with appropriate rise in salary and post-certificate training.

A structure for the administration of a service is shown in *Figure 4*. The ultimate responsibility for this service lies with the matron, who delegates it accordingly. Each section of the service has its own function – administration, teaching, and staffing of wards and departments.

Figure 5 depicts the supply of staff to the ward as a working unit. The ward unit is the meeting-point where the objectives of the hospital, i.e. treatment, training, and research, are carried out. The service provides staff for the wards and the staff are responsible through the line of control to the ward sister, who is responsible to the doctor. She carries out instructions, organizes the work, co-ordinates every aspect of the patients' requirements and ward care, supervising the nursing of the patient and the training of the student nurse.

FIGURE 4 A structure for the administration of a service

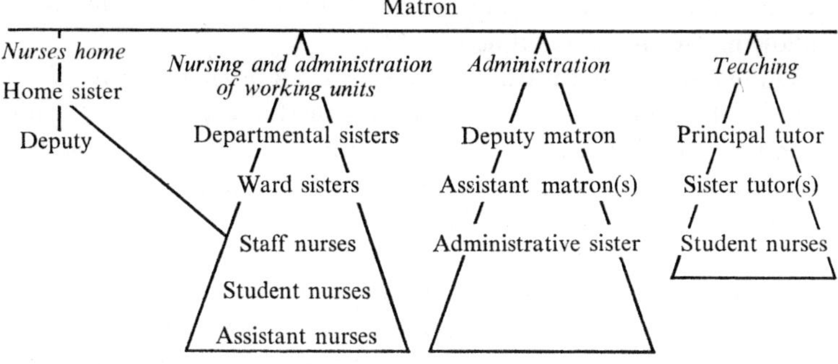

FIGURE 5 The supply of staff to the ward unit

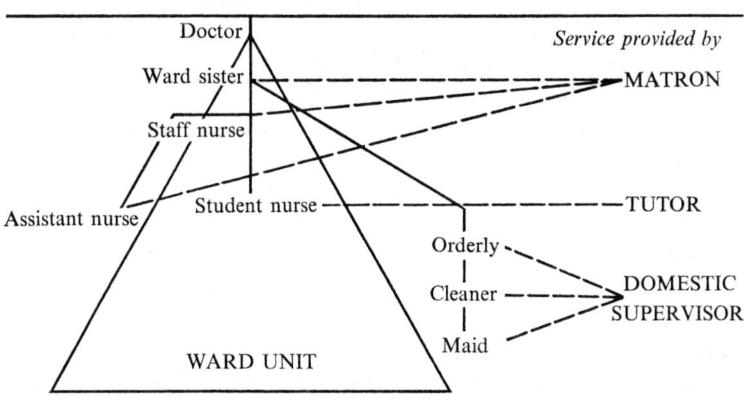

SOME PROBLEMS OF HOSPITAL STRUCTURE

Conflicting loyalties

The fact that the hierarchy is used to structure both the systems of seniority and the line of authority frequently causes confusion to the employee who is uncertain 'who is responsible to whom and for what'. It can be seen from the diagrams that each hierarchy is not separate and self-contained but at some point comes into contact with another, i.e. there are various points at which members of one hierarchy are responsible not only to a senior member of their own hierarchy but also to a member of another or partly so. For example, the sister is responsible to both the doctor and the matron, the ward cleaner is responsible to both the domestic supervisor and the sister. Many difficulties stemming from this situation were encountered in practice during the course of the investigation, as the following two incidents illustrate.

On one occasion a ward maid was in tears because she had been told by the domestic supervisor to put the buckets on the balcony after use, and by the ward sister to put them under the sink because the matron would not have the balcony cluttered up.

On another occasion a head porter had been told to make arrangements for the centralization of all oxygen cylinders, leaving only one small emergency cylinder on each ward. When the ward porter went to collect them in he was greeted by angry ward sisters who 'did not see why the porter should run the ward'. The battle raged between the ward sister and the head porter through the ward porter, with the result that he became unco-operative and noisy when wheeling the cylinders on to the ward, which in turn contributed to the noise disturbing the patients.

A further cause of confusion is seen in that each person has within himself a number of roles at one and the same time. For example, the sister is administrator, nurse, and teacher, and each role involves a relationship with a number of people, the matron, the doctor, and the tutor. One person may be responsible to two or more people even in the same hierarchy; thus a student nurse is responsible to both the sister and the tutor. To disentangle the resulting complex network of relationships is difficult, yet this confusion may contribute largely to interpersonal difficulties between members of the ward team and between the ward and the hospital. An example was seen in one hospital where the night nurse knew that the patients must not be called before 6 a.m. If she called them earlier and was caught by the night sister she would be reprimanded, but if the ward work was not complete for the day sister she would also be in trouble. The result was a furtive and guilty attempt to bath a patient by torch light, which proved to be an uncomfortable experience for the patient and an awkward task for the nurse.

Departmental thinking

This is both a cause and an effect of specialization and poor relationships. The department concentrates its attention on its own function, with little thought for the policy of the hospital as a whole. This is a natural reaction to shortage of staff and pressure of absorbing work, both often found in the ward unit. The isolation tends to lower the effectiveness of the hospital as a whole.

Scapegoating

Scapegoating may occur in certain types of department and may cause the staff to withdraw and become unhelpful. It is not uncommonly seen in the relationship of the stores to the hospital. Often, owing to shortage of supplies, financial pressure, or red tape, goods are delayed in reaching the appropriate ward or department. Irate telephone calls produce little results and the stores staff are held in disfavour through no fault of their own.

Prestige

Certain types of work carry more prestige than others, either through social convention or through a feeling that certain kinds of work are more worth while than others. This creates barriers between groups.

Non-mixing of groups

The groups within the departments themselves tend not to mix. This may occur, for example, in the nursing group with student nurses of different years. Even on the permanent staff, social mixing of the matron and the sisters is uncommon. Yet another source of difficulty is the split between the staff who cover a twenty-four hour span of duty in direct contact with the patient and those who have evenings and week-ends free. The former group consists predominantly of medical and nursing staff whose living arrangements, geared to meet irregular hours, tend to create an artificial barrier between them and the outside world. The latter are more aware of the hard realities of living in the form of travelling and housing problems, and are consequently more able to appreciate the kinds of problem patients have to face when they return home.

WARD ADMINISTRATION

The ward unit has been considered as part of the hospital with reference to the objectives of the hospital, the historical development of the hospital system, and its place in the national health service. Consideration is now given to the basic needs of the ward, ward management and its problems, and the organization of ward work.

BASIC NEEDS

The needs of the patient have already been referred to. Another important aspect is the provision of facilities for the visiting of the patient by his relatives and friends, for, despite more frequent visiting in many hospitals, the patient is still cut off from his family, sometimes unnecessarily. Each phase of illness has to be considered and thought has to be given to the patient who is not acutely ill, for his needs are frequently submerged in the interests of the smooth running of the ward as a whole. Increasing significance is given to the rehabilitation of the patient to work and home, and it may prove necessary ultimately to modify ward administration to meet these changing ideas.

Nursing staff need good training and working conditions, amenable off-duty, well-organized work, and opportunity fully to experience the satisfaction to be derived from caring for sick human beings. The problem of meeting and balancing various needs is greatly complicated by the perpetual state of change. Not only do both patients and staff move at varying but rather frequent intervals, but provision must be made for recurrent emergencies, changing demands on staff, and twenty-four-hour staffing.

WARD MANAGEMENT

Internal structure of the ward

The ward team and structure have been described as being based on a hierarchical framework which unifies the ward as a whole. At the same time it lends itself to the formation of a set of rules and regulations for the staff and is a useful structure for administration. The ward structure serves a purpose similar to that of the army structure by protecting staff, defining leadership, and giving sanction for the performance of tasks which may be unpleasant and hurtful to the patient. The role and function of each person in the face of danger can be strictly defined to allow for prompt action, each person falling into his proper place in the team performing the appropriate task. Finally, the structure creates a sense of security for the patient, defining his place and his relation with the staff. It serves as a useful framework within which to organize the routine of the ward irrespective of the people who are continually changing and passing through.

The ward team is headed by the sister, who is frequently the only permanent person in the ward. The rest of the nursing team stay from a few weeks to months and are then moved. In some hospitals the staff nurse is appointed for a period of six months to a year, and at times domestic staff stay on one ward for long periods. The ward sister has to co-ordinate the people in the ward and organize their work. She has to delegate much of the work to others.

Problems of ward management

Difficulties arise where shortage of staff and changing personnel make it hard to relinquish tasks for external reasons. At the same time, the ward sister may be reluctant to delegate responsibility to others because of a distrust of others' capabilities, which may be founded on reality. She may be governed by her own need to control everything herself. This is accentuated by her deep feeling of responsibility for the patients.

The word 'hierarchy' has become associated with autocratic rather than democratic behaviour and the criticism is made that the hierarchy is to blame for many of the ward tensions and problems. In fact, the hierarchy itself is only a structure useful for organizing staff for reasons already given. The behaviour within the hierarchy is very often autocratic, especially in crisis situations where orders must be obeyed quickly and without question. The need for absolute obedience then carries over into non-crisis situations. The effect of this is to militate against two-way discussion of problems relating to work, the pattern being set as a one-way communication. When emotions such as anger are aroused, human nature being what it is, it may be passed on rather than controlled. The well-known army story of the colonel kicking the major, the major the captain, and so on down the line until the soldier kicked the cat, is a good analogy. Unfortunately the 'soldier' may be the junior nurse and the 'cat' the patient. One patient said, 'We patients always watch sister's face in the morning as she walks on duty. If she is unsmiling we lie very still until she does smile, for her mood sets the mood of the staff and patients as a whole.'

Everyone working in this framework has certain problems connected with management and leadership, e.g. being managed, reacting to authority, and feeling excessive responsibility, some of which will be discussed below.

Management and leadership: The hierarchy puts the ward sister in the role of leader and manager of the whole unit. Her behaviour will be governed by external circumstances and internal feelings based on past experience. If the ward is busy, staff short, and demands heavy, she may attempt to control the ward and her own raised anxieties by autocratic behaviour. She may model her attitude on other more senior members of the staff, for example, the matron. It is often said that the way in which the matron copes with similar situations sets the pace and the pattern for her staff. This goes straight down the line, for the staff nurse takes her attitude from the ward sister and the nurses from the staff nurse. A calm leader prevents panic and confusion by her example. At the same time the sister is an individual with past experiences. The saying 'the child is father to the man' reminds one that the past is within each person and patterns of behaviour have often been formed in childhood and may still influence, to some extent, adult life and modes of behaviour. Furthermore, past nursing training and experience influence the present attitude to authority.

Being managed: The principles above apply to the subordinates. Overwork, shortage of staff, lack of experience and knowledge, may make the nurse too anxious, clumsy, slow, or apathetic. Her reactions to authority may be realistic, or past influence may make her unnecessarily angry or resentful when she is told what to do.

Feeling responsible: If the staff are to participate effectively, each person must know what to do and the amount of responsibility she has to take. In addition, she needs the appropriate authority to fulfil that responsibility. Responsibility for the work is split up as is the work itself. Problems arise when the person feels responsible for the set task but not for the task in relation to others. The task itself may be well done but, if the nurse does not recognize her responsibility to the ward team, the resulting lack of flexibility causes the work as a whole to suffer.

A common source of difficulty is that staff may feel responsible for a situation when, in fact, they are not so responsible. For example, the ultimate responsibility for the patient always lies with the doctor. The consultant, in his absence, delegates this to registrar or houseman. The sister who is on the spot often *feels* responsible when faced with a critically ill patient, especially when the houseman is young and inexperienced.

ORGANIZATION OF WARD WORK

Prevalence of job-assignment method

Out of fifty-seven wards, fifty-five used the job-assignment method of organizing their work. The sister divides the nursing of the patients and the ward work into groups of jobs and delegates these to the staff nurse and student nurses according to the woman/man power available at the time. The senior nurse performs skilled technical procedures, the junior nurse routine duties such as washing, feeding, and toilet rounds, and the 'middle' nurse fluctuates between the two. Each nurse reports to the sister, verbally or in writing, the results and observations made during the performance of these tasks. The sister brings together all the observations and reports to the doctor on his round. In this way the work of the ward as a whole is covered in a routine fashion governed by the clock.

Problems deriving from this method

For the patient: The patient is disturbed frequently by different people performing different tasks at different times. For example, he may have his bed made by one person, his back rubbed by another, and an injection given by somone else. If, in addition, the number of staff concerned with diagnosis and treatment is taken into account, it is obvious that he is attended to by many people. This is not only physically but mentally disturbing, because it takes energy to make relationships. The patient makes many superficial contacts but none of any depth. In such a situation, few of the staff develop a sense of personal responsibility for the patient as a person. The patient is thus deprived of opportunity to voice his personal affairs and anxieties; consequently, he is deprived of the reassurance necessary for his total recovery. Even the sister, who has the most complete picture of the patient, frequently uses her 'rounds' to inquire after the state of his bowels. It is not possible for her to make a real relationship with every one of thirty patients in the ward. One patient who was interviewed said, 'I had a minor dental operation so my stay in hospital lasted only five days. During that time I received excellent surgical treatment but I was left with the impression that I was only a mandible bone and a ration book to the staff.' He had been unable to discover 'to whom he could talk' on the staff, because he did not know which was the sister in charge of the ward until his last day.

This method of division of labour and job breakdown is commonly used in industry. The system has much to recommend it where the raw material is inanimate and the end-result an object. It leaves much to be desired when the work is concerned with people and the end-result is a changed person; for example, a sick person cured.

For the staff: The nurse is responsible for groups of jobs rather than people. Work-loads are heavy and, in order to complete her work for the ward sister in the given space of time, each nurse has to organize her activities with this as her primary aim rather than consideration for the comfort of the patient. The nurse becomes proficient and quick in the performance of nursing procedures. It would be impossible to do otherwise when, for instance, a nurse has to give ten injections every few hours, but she does not learn fully to appreciate the application of the procedure to and its effect on the patient and his disease.

The nurse is so busy trying to complete her work in a given time that she has no time to make a relationship with the patient which would help him and enable her to practise the real art of nursing. She is not encouraged to stop and talk to the patient – 'time is too valuable to waste'. A nurse could help more if she looked after patients rather than jobs. Many nurses start their careers with enthusiasm and a desire to help others. This is too often dampened by the performance of repeated jobs in the interests of the 'ward as a whole', but not for people as individuals. The high wastage of student nurses in the first year (Ministry of Health, 1948) may have as one of its causes the way in which the work is organized. Instead of utilizing the nurses' initial warmth and interest in people, it tends to dampen these and substitutes a more brittle set of values of efficiency and speed.

If the work is organized into groups of jobs, promotion is often felt by the nurse to be in terms of advancing from unskilled to skilled work. Unpleasant jobs are usually relegated to newcomers in any sphere of work, but in nursing these tasks are often vitally important to patient and doctor. If the nurse feels it degrading to return to 'junior' work, thus apparently lowering her prestige, her attitude affects the patient and the standard of nursing as a whole. Job assignment puts the trained nurse in a peculiar position. If work is divided into groups of junior, middle, and senior work, and the staff nurse deputizes for the sister, there is room only for one trained nurse in the ward. The second staff nurse has to do work she was doing as a senior nurse. This may make for discontent. It may also be one factor contributing to the present acute shortage of trained staff nurses, now that the four-year contract has been reduced to three years and the choice lies with the nurse as to whether or not she will stay after qualifying.

A great deal of very detailed planning and organization of work and time is necessary for the sister, who is the only person with an overall view of the ward or of any single patient. This method of detailed organization of tasks related to the total work of the ward splits up responsibility for the patient so that no one nurse has a picture of him as a whole person. This makes it difficult or impossible for her to relate her task to the whole patient or the whole illness, and to carry out this task against such a background. Only the sister has the complete picture and she has little to do with the actual nursing. The situation in which tasks are not carried out against the frame of reference of the patient as a whole person can easily lead to the situation in which they are carried out in a way that is detrimental to the patient.

It may also lead to tasks being carried out in a routine way, for each patient, despite the fact that there are important differences between patients. The nurse has little chance to appreciate these differences. Specific instructions to treat patients differently may easily be forgotten when the nurse gets into the swing of a routine task, as the following example shows. A patient suffering from a rare disease had to have all her urine saved to be tested by the laboratory technicians. Every precaution was taken by the ward sister, who was an excellent administrator. Instructions were written in the report book and on special lists. The nurses were told at report-time the reason for the saving of the urine and emphasis was placed on the importance of this factor for the patient and her diagnosis. Instructions were handed to the night staff in the report and in writing and yet the urine was thrown away. The patient's diagnosis and treatment were delayed, the nurses were filled with remorse, and the sister was upset and angry that her painstaking care should be thwarted in this way. It is true that the link between day and night staff is often weak but, if one nurse had been responsible for the whole patient, she, as well as the sister, would have felt a personal responsibility and would have understood better why these instructions were necessary.

The nurse tends to see her job and its effect in isolation. For example, a junior nurse carrying out a toilet round will quickly learn to distinguish abnormal from normal urine because she sees so many specimens. She is less likely to learn the significance of a normal or an abnormal specimen of urine in relation to the patient as an individual, or what her observations mean in terms of the patient's disease and treatment.

Each nurse observes a bit of each patient and reports this to the sister. The sister puts together the bits and translates them into a picture of each patient to tell the doctor. The sum total of the bits may not give the dynamic whole. An instance of this was seen in a ward where the staff nurse was told to give all the injections as part of her morning's work. She gave them speedily and efficiently but was delayed, and had one left to do as the lunches were beginning to be served. Rather than incur the sister's displeasure she went to a patient suffering from ulcerative colitis just as his lunch was placed before him. She apologized for disturbing him and asked if she might give the injection; he looked annoyed but said, 'Yes'. He ate very little lunch and later in the day developed a severe attack of diarrhoea. The reports given to the doctor read, 'The patient had his injection with no reaction. He ate very little lunch. He developed diarrhoea.' The diet was blamed and not the patient's unexpressed anger, which might have been a likely cause of relapse; it was not reported because not observed, falling between the two responsibilities. If one nurse had given the injection and the meal, and reported the total situation, a more accurate picture would have been given to the doctor.

The above example also shows the close link between the physical and mental state of the patients. It demonstrates, too, the inability of the patient to refuse the injection and the inability of the staff nurse to face the sister not having carried out her allotted task.

TRAINING IN THE WARD

TEACHING METHODS

Just as the efficiency and usefulness of the whole hospital administration are tested out in the ward, so, too, the efficiency of the training system comes out in the practical work with the patient. During the teaching of nursing procedure, the nurse is shown how to prepare equipment, prepare the patient, understand the technique employed, and perform the procedure on the patient. Having done this she notes the effect and reports verbally or in writing. Teaching in the classroom helps her to acquire basic knowledge about disease, the preparation of equipment, the technique of the nursing procedure and the possible effect on the patient, leaving her free to concentrate on its practical application to the patient when in the ward.

Although the student nurse learns the theory and practice of nursing in the classroom from the tutor, together with an understanding of symptoms of diseases and their treatment, and of certain aspects of the patient's behaviour, she needs help from an experienced person in the practical application of this knowledge to the patient in the ward. The ward is a busy place where the pressure of work may be such that the ward sister has little time to undertake the important function of teaching the student nurse.

Informal teaching

Informal teaching takes place in three main ways: by example, through supervision, and by good work organization.

Example: A good deal of learning takes place through the example of others. The ward sister sets the tone of the ward. The way she behaves, the way she works or deals with both well and ill people, has the greatest influence on the student nurse especially in her first year. What is important to the sister will become important to the student nurse and in this way 'good' or 'bad' habits are started. If the sister sees the patient predominantly as a case, so will the student nurse. The phrase, 'sister likes it that way', so often used by the staff, serves to demonstrate the significance of teaching by example. If this can be supplemented by the ward sister's putting into words what she is doing, why and how, as she goes about the ward, and if she is aware of the benefit the staff receive by this effort on her part, then valuable teaching opportunities will be used. Also, the student nurse will be trained to do the same in relation to junior student nurses.

Supervision: The everyday supervision of the student nurse by sister, staff nurse, or other senior nurse can be used as a teaching experience. If supervision is too strict the student nurse, through fear, will be unable to learn from her mistakes. If it is too slack a valuable opportunity will be lost to help the nurse to learn not only a good standard of nursing but what she is doing and why. Even minor mistakes in work may raise the student nurse's sense of guilt beyond proportion to the reality, especially where she feels her responsibility to the patient deeply. When the sister shows sympathy and understanding with the young nurse's difficulties when first dealing with the patients, she is generally repaid by the student nurse's gaining assurance and self-confidence which, in turn, are transmitted to the patient and add to his security.

Organization of work: This is one of the major factors contributing to the teaching in the ward. The organization reflects what is really considered to be of importance in practice in the ward. The effects of job assignment can at this point be considered in relation to training needs. This method of work trains the nurse to become proficient in technical nursing procedures and the organization of the work of the ward as a whole, and it teaches her to take responsibility for jobs rather than people. It has the effect of training her to be efficient, quick, and expert in physical nursing but it stunts her capacity for understanding the patient and relating nursing theory and practice to the patient, his background, and his disease. In other words, it prevents nursing in the widest sense, the complete care of the patient.

Formal teaching

Opportunities used by the ward sister for formal instruction vary according to the ward. They include ward reports, classes and practical demonstrations, and individual tuition.

Ward reports: The ward report occurs at the meeting of staff as they are relieved of or take over duty. The people who must attend the report are the person in charge (i.e. sister, senior night nurse, or staff nurse) and the person who will be in charge of the ward for the next few hours. Custom varies considerably from ward to ward and hospital to hospital as to which other members of the staff attend. In some wards all the staff collect at one point of the day to hear an account of the previous twenty-four hours' progress of the patients. But in many wards the most junior nurses never hear a report and gain their information from records and from inquiries from other nurses; it is not uncommon to find nurses not knowing what is the matter with the patients in the ward. From a teaching and a practical point of view it would appear essential that nurses of all grades, especially the junior nurse, should understand what is the matter with the patient. The report can be a useful teaching opportunity where, if time permits, the sister asks questions of the student nurse and vice versa.

Classes and practical demonstrations: Formal teaching of the student nurse varies according to the sister's interest and the work of the ward. Sometimes the sister or the staff nurse demonstrates preparation of equipment and carrying out of nursing procedure on a patient, with one or more nurses watching. The nurses then take turns to perform the nursing procedure either immediately afterwards or at a suitable time in the ward routine. Some sisters hold a formal class on a variety of topics such as the nursing of special diseases in the ward, or an account of a disease in relation to anatomy, physiology, signs and symptoms, and treatment. Case conferences on one or more patients may also be held. These classes take place at regular intervals or spasmodically, according to the individual sister.

PROBLEMS IN WARD TEACHING

For the ward sister, care of the patient is a more important and urgent responsibility than teaching. It is easy for her to forget that her nurses are students as well as ward staff, to forget her responsibility for teaching or to minimize its value. The student nurse may become involved in the urgency of nursing her patients and forget that part of her total responsibility is to learn. Many sisters give up the attempt to teach because of constant interruptions while trying to do so. One ward sister described an attempt to demonstrate to student nurses the giving of an injection. She had no fewer than ten interruptions during the three-minute demonstration. While this serves as a good example of the frequent demands made on the ward sister, it also demonstrates the low priority of teaching in relation to other aspects of ward work.

The division between classroom teaching and practical work often expresses itself in the student nurse's standard of practical nursing. The tutor teaches the 'correct' technique using the right equipment in the classroom. The nurse who is rushed for time, with possibly less equipment on the ward, may scamp the procedure with the result that there is one standard for the tutor and examinations and another for practical nursing in the ward. This situation may be reflected in strained relations between the tutor and the ward sister, each having difficulty in appreciating the other's point of view. These strained relations may also make things very difficult for the student nurse who has to please both at different times.

Different doctors may have differing opinions concerning the treatment of the same condition. This is inevitable with changing medical knowledge but it contributes to the difficulties of the student nurse who cannot grasp the principle or the sense in apparently conflicting treatments. At these times she has to trust blindly and use faith!

The demand of the teaching programme that the nurse should gain wide experience in nursing a variety of cases necessitates frequent changing from ward to ward. This means a break in old relations with staff and patients, a building of new cases, and adaptation to a new sister and doctor with different attitudes and routines. The result may be a feeling of insecurity and anxiety, which does not help learning. The nurse may find herself on a ward without having learned the appropriate theory or she may take her examinations without having practised the theory as taught in the classroom.

TRENDS IN HOSPITAL ADMINISTRATION

Specialization of large staffs has highlighted the need for co-ordination and co-operation. Many hospitals are trying to solve some of their difficulties by providing opportunities for people to meet and discuss problems formally as well as informally. Three main types of procedure are employed: joint consultative committees, interdepartmental meetings, and departmental meetings. During the course of this investigation, material was collected concerning the value of staff meetings and the methods used to conduct them. An analysis of the reasons for their success or failure, as seen by the staff concerned, is given below.

JOINT CONSULTATIVE COMMITTEES

National Whitley Council

This is a national body, set up to:

(i) enable all who work in the service to improve its efficiency;
(ii) provide a channel for the consideration of sectional claims and the remedying of grievances;
(iii) give speedy decisions on questions at issue and ensure co-ordination through the service.

Committees of the Council are made up of representatives of nationally accepted employing authorities and staff organizations, and arrive at their decisions by a process of negotiation.

Joint consultative staffs committees

These committees are set up in each hospital. Membership of a committee consists of certain members of the hospital management committee or board of governors, known as the management side, and elected representatives of the staff groups, i.e. administrative and clerical staff, nursing and midwifery staff, technical and professional staff (other than nurses and midwives), domestic, farm, garden, and artisan staff, always provided that the persons elected shall be members of a nationally recognized negotiating body. The committee meets at regular intervals and has as its functions:

'To promote the closest co-operation and provide a recognized means of consultation between the management committee or board of governors, its senior officers and staff.

To give the staffs a wider interest in and a greater responsibility for the conditions under which their work is performed; to give the maximum assistance in promoting the welfare of the patients and efficient administration in the hospitals controlled by the committee or board; to make suggestions for the improvement of the general arrangements for the comfort of the staff, their recreation, entertainments and dietary.

To prevent friction and misunderstanding.

Subject to the proviso that no recommendations of the hospital staffs committee shall conflict with, or override, any decision of the general council or the appropriate functional council, to deal with such matters as:

(i) the distribution of working hours;
(ii) holiday arrangements;
(iii) questions of physical welfare – cloakroom arrangements, heating, ventilation, etc.

To consider any hospital rules affecting staff, apart from any that may be prescribed nationally or regionally.'[1]

INTERDEPARTMENTAL MEETINGS

Within the nursing group two main types of meeting were seen: staff meetings and nursing procedure committees.

Staff meetings

All but two of the hospitals studied held meetings between the matron and the permanent nursing staff. Interviews with matrons and sisters produced a divergence of opinion as to whether or not these meetings were of value. In four hospitals both the matron and the sisters found the meetings useful; in one hospital neither the matron nor the sisters considered them helpful; in six hospitals the matron felt that they served a limited purpose but the sisters regarded them as a waste of time; in one hospital the matron judged

[1] Whitley Councils for the Health Services (Great Britain). General Council. General Council Circular No. 20.

them of little value but the sisters liked them. The remainder of the hospitals either thought they had not tried the meetings long enough or volunteered no opinion. The hospitals finding staff meetings to be of value had all given considerable thought to the aims and structure of such meetings. Certain points of aim and structure will be discussed below.

The size of the meetings varied from thirty to a hundred people, depending on the size of the hospital and the types of staff invited. In one hospital, in order to make the meetings more manageable, the matron divided the staff so that ward sisters and staff nurses attended on one occasion, and departmental sisters and staff nurses on another. The majority of hospitals, however, called administrative staff, ward and departmental sisters, tutors, home sisters, and staff nurses to the one meeting. In the author's opinion, meetings of so large a number make it difficult to ensure adequate discussion of problems. Moreover, the choice of a method of conducting such meetings is limited by their size. The most useful procedure would appear to be a more formal one, with a chairman (who may or may not be the matron) following the agenda closely and leaving time at the end of the meeting for discussion.

The length of the staff meetings and the frequency with which they were called varied also. In some hospitals a meeting was called 'if matron has anything to say', averaging two or three times a year. One hospital held a weekly meeting straight after lunch, but the majority of hospitals held monthly meetings which all staff were expected to attend, however busy. One meeting started informally with tea, and the business meeting immediately followed. Meetings varied from ten minutes to one hour in length. Matrons held different opinions on this matter: some felt that a full hour should be taken whether the meeting was used or not; whereas others considered a few minutes ample, any additional time being time wasted.

The four hospitals in which both the matron and the sisters found staff meetings useful were agreed on the point that, although the agenda was compiled by the matron, it should be possible for anyone to add to it, and that the agenda should be circulated in advance so that all the staff could consider it. Pinning the agenda on the staff board did not seem to be as effective as individual circulation, though the latter method was more extravagant in paper and time. Some hospitals did not advertise the agenda in advance but simply notified the staff of the time of the meeting.

A good deal of confusion appears to exist as to the terms of reference of the staff meeting. The vague term, 'to discuss staff problems', does not seem to be clear enough. The lack of definition of the relationship between the nursing service as a whole and the working unit, with its confusion of responsibilities, was demonstrated by discussion at staff meetings of some issues that should have been discussed in the working unit with the doctor if opportunity had been made. That is, the meetings were used as a 'dust-bin' for problems that could not be solved elsewhere. Such meetings may allow for blowing off steam but are not always followed by constructive action. Questions that might usefully be discussed in a staff meeting could include those relating to training, nursing techniques, and standards of nursing, together with domestic matters concerning the nursing staff as a whole. Staff meetings may also be used for passing on relevant material from other departments and from management committees in the interest of the hospital as a whole. The meetings would thus serve two main functions: in the first place, acting as a 'briefing' or informative meeting, with the matron telling the staff various points of universal interest; in the second place, providing an opportunity for the discussion of specific nursing problems. After discussion of a topic, a decision may be reached. The next step is to secure its implementation. The decision may be expressed in the form of a recommendation *advising* action or of a recommendation with authority to give an *order* to act. Confusion frequently arises as to whether the recommendation is advisory or executive.

It is impossible to consider what use such meetings may be to the staff concerned without thinking of the individual people who attend them and the background against which the meetings take place. Perhaps the essential ingredient for a useful meeting is a real sincerity on all sides that it should serve a good purpose. Some meetings were described as being apathetic and silent, with comments such as 'it's no use talking'; 'matron only says "no"'; 'nothing happens anyway'; 'it's a waste of time'. At the other extreme meetings were described as active, productive, and 'a real opportunity to work as a team'. The former descriptions might be considered as 'symptoms' reflecting that the meetings had not been constructed well and/or that the staff did not really want to get together in the first place. There are other causes, some of which will be examined below.

The meeting often tends to mould itself on the pattern of the hierarchy, in which the matron is the senior person. Where two-way discussion is needed it is difficult to forget this factor, so that the matron does the talking rather than the staff, and her position prevents them from saying what they think. Not only is the matron the employer and the staff the employees, but discussions of a critical nature on any issue may be felt to jeopardize the security of a job or a chance of promotion. At the same time, the traditional interpretation of the one-way system influences the actions of the staff. They still do not feel free to speak and participate as colleagues of the matron, with a common aim. Anything the matron might say tends to be interpreted as an order rather than as a comment or advice, which the staff may or may not adopt as they think fit.

Silence and apathy often indicate unexpressed hostility. The hostility may have a real origin in that the sisters dislike the matron, but it is more probable that it is based on traditional attitudes regardless of the individual. The hostility may be displaced from the working unit or it may represent a reaction to authority.

Whatever the real or fancied difficulties may be, staff meetings will go through a period of growing pains before settling down. It is difficult to step out of long-accustomed attitudes and roles and recognize that a meeting of the matron and the staff can really be of value. A pattern frequently seen is, first of all, a testing out of the sincerity of the matron to prove that she really means that problems can be discussed and critical thoughts voiced when necessary. The next stage may produce a storm of complaints, often about food, or difficulties with doctors, and requests are made that matters be put right. This can be a trying time for both sides: for the staff because they are disillusioned, wanting action, not talk; for the matron because she is annoyed that the staff are unable to see that she is powerless to alter many things. Finally, with perseverance, it is possible to work through to a more mature situation where staff and matron contribute their experiences to the finding of common solutions of mutual benefit through discussion. To achieve this a certain amount of frustration has to be tolerated on both sides.

Nursing procedure committees

These are small committees composed of the matron, tutors, and ward and departmental sisters. They are set up for the purpose of discussing nursing procedures and to ensure the integration of classroom and ward teaching.

Thirteen hospitals had procedure committees, and six of these expressed the opinion that they were of value. Although many of the points considered above apply to the procedure committee meeting, there are certain differences. With regard to size, procedure committee meetings are much smaller than staff meetings, therefore discussion can take place more easily. Their aims are clearly defined, and the members usually remain the same except that a specialist sister may be called in to discuss special nursing techniques. Where the results of the procedure committee were good, it would appear that careful consideration had been given to the working through and implementation period. The recommendations of the committee were taken to the staff meeting and discussed. If the staff did not agree with them they were referred back to the committee until a unanimous decision was reached. To achieve implementation, the ward sisters informed the nurses in their wards of the agreed recommendations, the tutors taught them in the classroom, and the matron reported them to the representative student nurses' committee. The recommendations were also printed and circulated in a loose-leaf file kept in an easily accessible place, and the procedure was reviewed and, if necessary, changed as treatments changed.

The co-operation of matron, tutors, and ward sisters in the procedure committee can have a valuable influence. Not only is the standard of nursing raised, but the uniformity of the basic nursing procedures helps to minimize the anxiety felt by the student nurse as she moves from ward to ward, and the patient receives more consistent treatment. Although there still remain differences between classroom and ward practice, and there are differences between the wards in respect of time schedules and the quality and quantity of available equipment, the procedure committee brings to light some of the problems, and provides an opportunity for finding solutions. Whether or not the opportunity is used depends – as with the staff meetings – on good organization, on a recognition of its importance, and on the desire that the committee's recommendations should be put into practice.

DEPARTMENTAL MEETINGS

At no time in any ward visited did all the staff meet together as a ward team to consider overall working problems. Subsections of the team met frequently during the formal ward round, the ward reports, and administrative reports.

Ward round

The doctors meet the sister to hear her observations, discuss and decide on the diagnosis and treatment of the patient, and issue the necessary instructions. Reference has already been made to the way in which these rounds are conducted, the senior doctor setting the example in his approach to the patient.

Ward reports

These serve a number of functions. They are used to pass on the instructions of the doctors to the staff in order that they may be carried out; to receive observations made by the staff concerning the patient, his condition and treatment; to hand over the ward to the next person in charge; to teach staff, if time and inclination permit; to pass on to staff relevant overall hospital matters and instructions from the matron. Attention has already been drawn to the fact that not all nursing staff receive a regular report. The practice would appear to vary not only from hospital to hospital, but from ward to ward in the same hospital, as to who attends while the report is given.

Administrative reports

Most wards are visited by a member of the nursing administrative staff once or twice a day. The night sisters are centralized in the matron's office and receive a report concerning the patient's condition from the nursing administrative staff, who have in turn received it from the ward sister, or the nurse in charge of the ward. The rest of the ward team are covered by the sister, who sees individual domestic staff and other people connected directly or indirectly with the welfare of the patients or ward.

MODERN METHODS OF MANAGEMENT AND INSTRUCTION OF STAFF IN INDUSTRY

SOME EFFECTS OF LARGE-SCALE PRODUCTION

Organizations other than hospitals have to face problems arising out of changing knowledge with resulting specialization of work and people and complex administration. In education, industry, and mining, for example, there has been a progressive splitting up of the task among more people, none of whom is any longer directly responsible for the whole task and its performance. Responsibility has now moved higher up the executive chain, to the headmaster, the foreman, and to the sister in nursing. These do not, as a rule, carry out the task. They organize the work of a group of people who perform the task among them. Detailed knowledge of the subjects in which student nurses receive instruction today is much greater than hitherto. This tends to create an attitude of specialization in such subjects and to discourage integration of related facts in the subjects taught.

Industry during the last two hundred years has developed from craft organizations, with a few workmen using their skill to complete set tasks, to large-scale mass-produced, machine-driven operations, with vast numbers of people doing one or two tasks only on a part of a finished product.

In the mining industry at one time, two or three men would complete all the necessary jobs, working together from start to finish. Their good teamwork was a necessity from the point of view of both work and safety. Today, many methods are in use, a common one being the working of a three-shift system with each shift completing a certain task so that the whole cycle of getting coal is completed in the twenty-four hours. This means that the whole process is never seen by any of the teams individually.

Where people worked in small groups, starting and finishing a piece of work, developing a pride in it and feeling responsible for it, knowing why and for whom the work was done, interpersonal relationships were worked out all the time on the job. Solutions to difficulties were based on tradition and face-to-face discussion. Practical training was carried out under the apprenticeship system where each stage of the job was learned over a period of years.

Today the large organizations, complex administrative machinery, specialization, while producing more and (sometimes) better goods, have also created many problems affecting the people who work in these organizations. The repercussions of the industrial revolution are still being felt – not in terms of work conditions, wages, and standards of living, for these have improved beyond recognition, but in other ways. Specialization has highlighted the necessity for co-ordination of work and co-operation of staff if production is to be maintained. It was well known in the Second World War that unity of purpose made many people work harder and longer than usual, for common danger binds people together. In peacetime this bond is relaxed and interpersonal difficulties come to the surface, assuming greater importance. If staff do not work well together, poor team spirit contributes to inefficiency, unhappiness, apathy, and minor ill health. Good team spirit, on the other hand, makes for happiness and a sense of wellbeing and satisfaction, which are reflected in competent vigorous work. To develop initiative, a sense of responsibility, and good teamwork, each person must know how to do his task in relation to others, his part in the team, and the relation of the team as a whole to the total organization. Some modern methods to achieve this will be discussed below.

DELEGATION OF AUTHORITY AND RESPONSIBILITY

One person can deal directly with only a certain number of people. This means that each working group must have a leader or foreman who in turn is responsible to someone else. Each link in the chain means that management becomes more remote and further away from the people doing the work. It is essential that each person should know to whom he is responsible and that he should be directly responsible to one person only. He needs to know, too, the bounds of his responsibility, whether it be for people working under him or for practical work.

The ability to administer is not the prerogative of the administrative staff at the top end of the scale. It may be found within each person whatever task he or she may be doing. It is the task of the administrator to see that each person is able to utilize his ability by delegating the requisite balance of responsibility and authority to meet the necessary work.

WORK ORGANIZATION

The organization of the work itself may take various forms. Where the task involves handling material, an attempt is being made to bring together groups of jobs for one person, rather than have one person doing one job all the time. Or, where the task is such that it cannot be added to others, staff are moved from job to job so that they learn a wider variety of tasks. Where the work involves dealing with people rather than material, the people are divided into groups so that one person is responsible for a smaller group rather than for certain aspects of a larger number of individuals. There are many spheres in which such measures are impracticable, but thinking people are realizing the importance of work organization and its relationship to staff morale and efficiency. Industry is now beginning to feel that the disadvantages of splitting up tasks may outweigh the advantages. A process of reintegration is beginning to take place in the most advanced fields of industry.

GROUP DISCIPLINE AND LEADERSHIP

Wherever a group of people work or live together there must be rules and discipline of two kinds, external and internal. External discipline consists of rules and regulations made by people other than the working group in the interests of the total organization. These rules and regulations must be kept. All organizations must have common rules of this nature but the fewer and more realistic they are the better, and the less likely they are to be broken. Each working unit has, in addition, its own rules, customs, and traditions. Current industrial practice is beginning to recognize that, if the person in charge makes the rules, and imposes them on the group without consultation, they are likely to be used as a weapon against authority and broken when possible. If, on the other hand, the group helps to make its own rules in consultation with the leader, it is more likely to keep them and to accept responsibility for them.

Each working unit has a leader who may be official or unofficial. The official leader is appointed by the employer in a foreman or manager role. The unofficial leader is chosen by the group for a variety of reasons but usually represents the *felt* interests of the working group. For example, a discontented group of men might produce an aggressive leader to speak for them. Or the leader might be a quiet unassuming man who lets others speak and encourages the expression of their views and ideas; his ability is to integrate and implement their wishes, and to help to develop the group as a whole. This may be the pattern of leadership necessary to achieve true democracy.

FORMAL AND INFORMAL COMMUNICATION

If staff are to work well with each other and take an active interest, not only in their own jobs but in the policy of the work group and the organization as a whole, it is necessary to provide opportunities for them to learn both local and general policy, to contribute to it, and to discuss work problems. Informal discussion while on the job, or during breaks, gives opportunity to settle many local differences of opinion, but more formal opportunities are required to bring to light problems of a wider nature. These formal channels of communication may be of four kinds – some of which have already been considered:

joint consultation, where conditions of service, wages, and general complaints are discussed in conjunction with trade unions;

general meetings, where overall problems of work are discussed and both administrative personnel and workers are invited to contribute their opinions to the broad policy of the works;

departmental meetings, where whole departments discuss problems concerned with their special aspect of the total task, e.g. finance;

local meetings of working groups, where day-to-day practical problems directly connected with the carrying out of the task are discussed.

SELECTION AND INDUCTION

Industry has recognized that it is useless to place a worker in a job for which he is unsuited, to place a man who is excellent at practical work in an administrative job unless he is able to assume leadership and deal with other people. To be good at one thing does not necessarily mean to be good at others and a 'square peg in a round hole' may have repercussions on other people. Good job placement is achieved by knowledge of the job, the work situation, and the man. Modern methods of selection assist in assessment of the man, but there is a danger of giving too much importance to these selection procedures. Industry often concentrates on improving the technique of selecting employees to avoid looking at the internal structure and functioning of the organization itself. This means that although time and money are spent in finding the right man, insufficient time and money are spent on assessing the job and the work situation. Where an unsatisfactory placement is made the selection methods are often blamed, whereas the real cause may be found in any one or all of the points, namely, in the worker, the job, the administration, or the work situation. If each aspect is not carefully studied a true balance cannot be reached.

The induction period for newcomers is important in any work. The newcomer has to learn not only how to do his job but many other things besides. He has to get to know his colleagues, the 'language' of the group, and its traditional customs. Most people find settling into a new job a strain and have different ways of dealing with it. They may react nervously, aggressively, or calmly; they may show their feelings or hide them. Whatever the newcomer's temperament, it is a stressful time for him. His discomfort can be reduced if he is 'shown the ropes' by a colleague or the person in charge, or attached to a member of the working group for a few days, even if he is provided with a pamphlet giving information on the policy, amenities, rules, and regulations of the firm.

Industry is groping towards a solution of the problems of specialization and reintegration with varying degrees of success. It is trying to return to the former satisfactions of craftsmanship without the disadvantages, but a good deal stands in the way. Perhaps first and foremost is human nature itself, resistant to change, suspicious of new ideas and attitudes, especially when past experience has proved painful. Where administrators genuinely believe in principles of democracy it is difficult for them not to be hurt and angry when their sincere intentions are thought to be insincere. If real development is to take place it will do so slowly, painfully, and with resistance.

Hospitals are facing similar problems but are in an even more difficult situation because they are dealing with people and the need to provide for recurrent emergencies instead of with inanimate material. It is easier to grumble against authority than to do anything about it, to hand responsibility on to someone else than to accept it squarely, and to blame others or the tools rather than oneself if the job goes wrong.

The principles outlined above aim at developing true self-government, which calls for maturity of the group as a whole and of the individuals in it. In this way the individual is encouraged to show initiative; he is able to derive satisfaction from his work, to develop a sense of responsibility, and to contribute to good relationships. The end-result should be a better standard of work.

CONCLUSIONS AND RECOMMENDATIONS

The hospital ward has been described in relation to the hospital as a whole – its objectives and history, and the administrative structure that has developed over the years. The main themes are:

1. The ward cannot be considered in isolation from the hospital, nor the hospital in isolation from society.

2. Changing medical knowledge has led to specialization of jobs and people with subsequent development of a large administrative structure giving rise to a new set of problems.

3. The structure of the hospital and training programmes have developed unevenly and have not always kept abreast of the times; this has led to difficulties of organization and confusion of responsibilities.

4. The breakdown of treatment into groups of tasks may lead to individual tasks being carried out efficiently and quickly but may result in less efficiency in carrying out the overall nursing task in relation to sick people, and in deeper repercussions on the patients and staff.

Some of the ways in which hospitals have attempted to meet these problems have been considered.

A brief survey was made of some of the practices employed in modern management and training in other organizations which are faced with similar problems of specialization and rapid change. In summary, it can be said that good management is dependent on:

1. Clear knowledge of structural organization, of the relationships to each other of the people working in the direct executive line, and of the relationships between that line and the various service units which assist in carrying out the total task.

2. Study and practice of modern methods of selection of staff.

3. Provision of opportunities for consultation, discussion of work problems, and participation in general policy.

4. Breakdown into small working groups, to allow development of leadership, individual initiative, responsibility, and good team spirit.

5. Especially when the work involves people, its breakdown into groups of workers rather than groups of jobs.

The application of these practices to ward administration is now discussed.

GENERAL OBSERVATIONS

Modern methods of management cannot be applied to ward administration without change in both the organizational structure of the hospital and the attitudes of its staff. Any significant change in organization at ward level will throw its relationship with the hospital out of gear unless corresponding changes are made throughout. For example, a change from job assignment to case assignment would be likely to necessitate certain changes in the work of the sister tutor and in the plan of practical work for student nurses, which, in turn, would affect the staffing arrangements.

Although other organizations have advanced further, in many ways, than hospitals in the recognition and attempted solution of problems of administration and management, their solutions cannot be transplanted unmodified to the hospital field. At the same time, some of the principles and practices employed in these other spheres could usefully be examined for their relevance to the hospitals' problems, so long as it is remembered that the end-results of industry are manufactured articles and profits from their sale, whereas hospitals deal with sick human beings.

This investigation has been a small-scale pilot study which has served to show up the great complexity of problems and the need for further work. The first and main recommendation is based on these general considerations.

Recommendation I: A full-scale investigation should be made in one hospital, to study its administration, relationships, and system of consultation, in the light of an evaluation of its objectives and needs. Such an investigation would be incomplete if it did not take into account the problems of introducing the necessary changes. It should go further, therefore, and the investigators should collaborate with the hospital in producing changes and studying their effects. This kind of investigation would be possible only in a hospital which itself recognized the need for, and was willing to undergo, the processes of change.

REPLANNING WARD ADMINISTRATION

To apply any of these principles of organization and management to a ward unit, certain basic requirements are necessary. First, the ward sister, whose task is to nurse, administer, and teach, must decide which of these functions she can most usefully delegate in the interests of the patients and the ward as a whole. If the concept of the patient's treatment already described is accepted, the need for case assignment is obvious. But case assignment can work well only where the nurse feels responsibility for and interest in the patient as a whole person. It is with these thoughts in mind that the second recommendation is made.

Recommendation II: The ward sister should delegate the nursing of the patients to the trained staff, and to student nurses under their supervision. There would thus be greater contact between the nurse in charge of the patient and the patient's doctor.

Recommendation III: (i) Trained nurses should be appointed to a ward for a period of six months to one year. (ii) Students should remain on one ward for from three to six months.

Emergencies such as staff sickness or a sudden change of ward inevitably occur. This paper has tried to show that delegation is impossible if the staff do not remain together long enough to develop as an autonomous group capable of taking responsibility. The implications of this recommendation are wide, since the nurse-training system usually in operation makes it necessary for staff to be moved frequently.

Recommendation IV: A centralized pool of relief nurses should be maintained as part of the training scheme.

Description of roles

A plan of ward administration based on these recommendations is shown in *Figure 6*, and its implications for the roles of ward personnel are noted briefly below.

FIGURE 6 Replanned ward administration

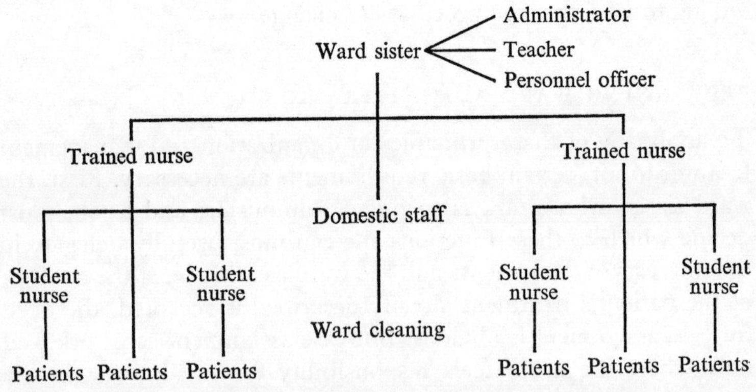

Ward sister: (*a*) administers the ward as a whole and acts as liaison between it and the hospital;

(*b*) co-ordinates small subgroups within the ward; all those concerned with domestic and maintenance work; all the staff involved with the patients, and the patients' relatives, but referring them to the appropriate nurse;

(*c*) develops personnel management role, paying particular attention to new staff and to problems of nursing resulting from the deeper contact between nurse and patient;

(*d*) teaches administration to trained nurses, nursing to student nurses, positive and preventive health to staff, patients, and relatives.

Trained nurses: (*a*) nurse patients;
(*b*) supervise nursing done by student nurses;
(*c*) learn overall administration from ward sister, acting in turns as her deputy;
(*d*) learn the practical application of management principles in dealing with a small group of staff.

Student nurses: (*a*) nurse patients under supervision:
(*b*) learn how to nurse, work in a team, and accept responsibility.

Domestic staff: clean ward and annexes under ward sister's supervision, and accept responsibility for these.

All subgroups would have allotted to them certain tasks, such as the tidiness of annexes or the maintenance of equipment. The relief nurse would need to be senior, to cover all grades of work.

General principles behind the plan

The basic principle is to divide the ward into units small enough to allow each to develop its natural resources to meet its own needs. The original grouping of doctor, patient, and nurse is repeated until the whole ward is covered on that basis.

Instead of the ward sister being the only person in the ward with an all-round view of the patients, each nurse would know a small number of the patients.

The most difficult administrative problems would be:

(*a*) keeping the ward sister informed of the patients' progress;
(*b*) co-ordinating the small units into the ward as a whole;
(*c*) meeting the extensive training requirements of the student nurses to ensure that they gained experience of a variety of nursing within the ward.

Their solution would depend in part on good informal relationships throughout the ward, and in part on a system of formal meeting-points which would regularly keep everyone up to date (see *Figure 7*).

FIGURE 7 System of ward meetings to co-ordinate administrative, teaching, and treatment objectives

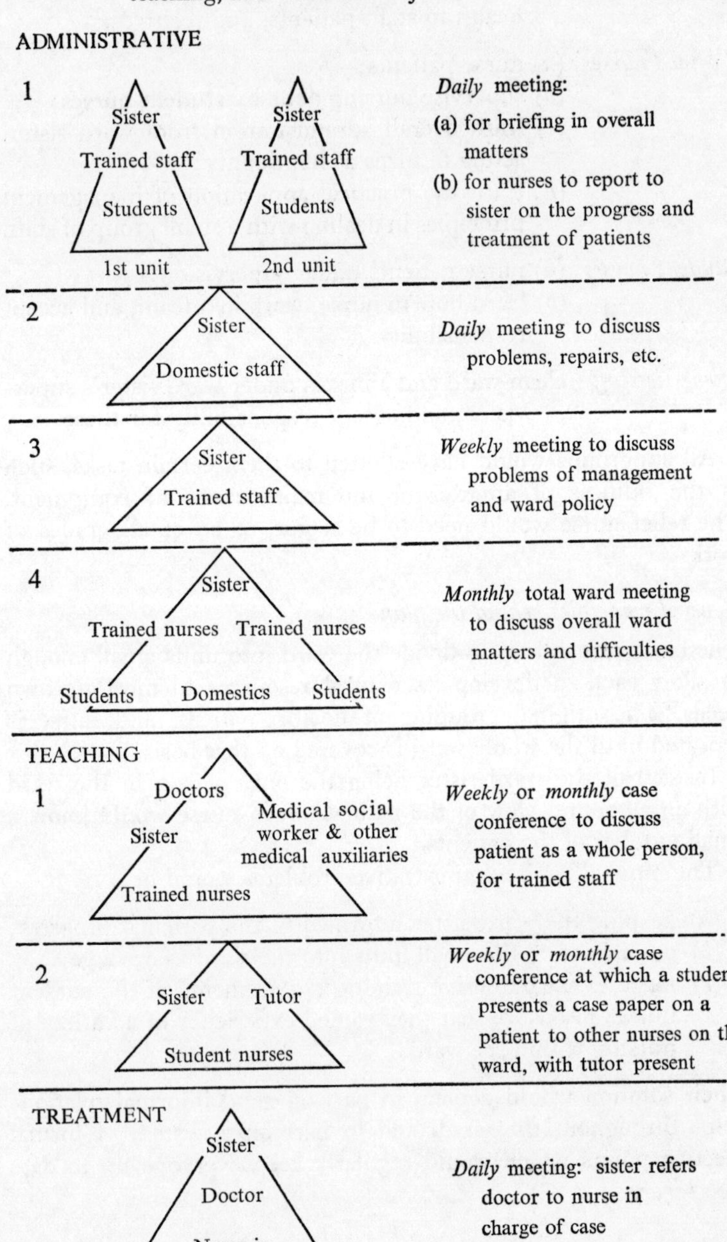

Both patients and staff should gain from a less centralized system of ward organization:

(*a*) the patient would be seen and treated as a whole person;

(*b*) the student nurse would have opportunity to relate nursing theory and practice to the patient as an individual, and would be allowed to use her capacity and enthusiasm for making relationships, which would help the patient and be more satisfying to herself;

(*c*) the trained nurse (other than the ward sister) would have a more satisfying role – nursing patients, learning how to supervise and teach students, and learning administration from the ward sister;

(*d*) the ward sister, although she might find her new role more frustrating at first in that she would not have the complete centralized control that she was used to, would have the satisfaction of knowing that each patient was better cared for and that the student nurses were receiving a more valuable training; moreover, the whole ward team would be sharing the responsibility which has hitherto fallen too heavily and exclusively on her shoulders.

27 · *Changing Hospital Attitudes*[1]

BY ELIZABETH BARNES

Public and professional discussion on how patients are treated in hospital is one of the more encouraging prominent features of the current scene in the United Kingdom's national health service. It exploded violently and with great heat in the medical, nursing, and general press, at conferences, and in board and committee rooms when Bowlby (1951) in print and Robertson (1953) on film first showed us what we were doing to children in hospital. Even today, nurses and doctors find 'good' reasons for keeping parents away from their hospitalized children. But official sanction from the Ministry of Health and the example of a few enlightened hospitals show a move towards the recognition that continuing the pattern of a child's life at home can be as necessary for medical treatment as it is for ordinary human development and that the latter can at times be the more important consideration. As Bowlby remarks: 'Fortunately, many of the less-developed countries have never forsaken this natural arrangement.'

The move, reluctantly, hedged with innumerable provisos and diluted with compromise, is now extending to the non-medical management of adult patients. For example, rules about visiting are being relaxed in most hospitals and dispensed with altogether in a few (Irvine & Smith, 1963). Ward routines are being revised to cut out ancient nursing rituals and thus give nurses more time to nurse in a wider sense, to hold ward meetings and educational discussions, and to give patients a more normal waking time and a rest in the afternoons (Ministry of Health, 1961). The grand round

[1] Based on a talk given at the Royal College of Nursing Southampton Branch Conference, held at Southampton University, September 1962; subsequently published in the *International Journal of Nursing Studies*, Vol. 1, pp. 11–16, 1963.

of the chief and his retinue is beginning to be seen as a quaint practice which insults the patient as a human being and teaches the medical student an archaic medical attitude. This move to make life in hospital more like life at home is an issue guaranteed always and perhaps unavoidably to arouse a highly emotional response, a curious mixture of censure and sentimentality.

The natural, untutored response to sickness and pain so great as to require hospitalization is fear. To counteract fear and in order to deal with its cause, the cultivated, tutored response must be one which will in all circumstances control it – by suppression if all else fails. Menzies (1960) describes some of the methods of control. The impersonalization of nursing, by non-attachment to patients, by splitting the total nursing care into a number of tasks performed by different nurses, by the implicit assumption that any patient or any nurse is the same as any other patient or nurse, avoids the stress and anxiety inherent in the job of nursing and reduces the burden of total responsibility. Menzies saw this as a 'social defence system [which] represented the institutionalization of very primitive defence mechanisms the main characteristic of which is that they facilitate the evasion of anxiety but contribute little to its true modification'. Such a system 'prevents true insight into the nature of problems and realistic appreciation of their seriousness'. The initial outraged reception accorded to this important paper merely underlined what Menzies uncovered. Much of her thinking has now passed into progressive nursing opinion.

We take complete control of our patients' lives because we take complete responsibility. We tend to suppress free expression of thought, feeling, and action in ourselves and our patients. We cannot allow the possibility of panic and disorder. We regulate our behaviour and attitudes to each other and to patients in order to create the kind of setting we feel is necessary for the work we have to do. Revans (1960) comments: 'No doubt the relation between doctor, nurse and patient is so apparently obvious that few have paused to ask precisely what it is, and upon what assumptions the existing systems of hospital organization are based; it may be that an ethic of clinical command, simple and austere, assuming as a natural law the immediate compliance of the subordinate, has for too long obscured the labyrinthine complexity of what in fact underlies effective co-operation in the hour of urgency.' Discussion which is both rational and investigatory about human relations in hospital and about efforts to 'humanize' hospital procedures becomes well-nigh impossible, it seems: on the one hand, because there is too much feeling, and, on the other, because there is too much control.

The essential question which those of us who indulge in this discussion are in danger of side-tracking is: What does a patient come to hospital for? He comes with some condition which, suddenly or slowly, has changed his life from health to sickness and he wants us to put it right. Essentially, then, his needs complement our own. Or, as Main (1963) puts it: 'Our response mirrors his need, and the more his distress the more concerned we become.'

Patients allow us to take them into hospital, put them to bed, find out what is wrong, try to put it right; and when we have done all we can we send them home. To do all this we know we shall have to cause further pain and discomfort. We shall have to cut them, stick in needles and tubes, make them swallow distasteful pills and liquids. We shall make them get up when they long to stay in bed and are sure they will never be able to set foot on the floor, or we shall make them stay in bed when they long to get up. They have to bear it all and we have to bear the feeling that we are hurting them and making them do things they would rather not. But we do these things, and they allow us to.

What we in fact do is to respond to the patients' first and essential need to get better. We take care of medical needs. We restore order where there was disorder, peace where there was panic. And we do this part of it very well.

But while we are dealing with medical needs we come up against other issues. We regulate and organize every other facet of patients' lives according to what we believe is best for them. We decide when they shall sleep, eat, wash, urinate, talk, read, listen to the radio. We even decide when they shall see their families. We have the power to separate husband from wife, parent from child, brother from sister, at a time of pain and stress when family members need each other. We remove the right of a normal man or woman to make decisions, even the smallest. We take it upon ourselves to judge all the patients' needs, thoughts, and actions while they are with us. And luckily for the peace of the ward and our self-confidence in the way we do things, they let us – usually without any protest. More often than not, they leave us full of praise and gratitude for what we have done. There is probably no other situation in life in which people hand themselves over, body and soul, completely and voluntarily – even gladly – to the ministrations of others.

Let us examine more closely the mutual attitudes of the people involved. First, what happens to us? The patient comes to us weak, frightened, and appealing for help. He sees us as strong, confident, and able to help. The weaker he feels the stronger he sees us. The more frightened he feels the more confident he sees us. In reality, what makes us strong and confident and gives us the ability to help is our training, experience, and skill. But human perception is based on more than reality; it is also phantasy, feeling, and imagination. One of the curiosities of human nature is that our perception is dominated and coloured more by phantasy than by reality when we are sick. The patient, who knows little of the realities of nursing, invests us with just these qualities of strength, power, and knowledge which he at this time needs to see in us. Have you ever watched a patient's face when he is looking at a doctor or a nurse? That typical cowed, stupefied look, the eyes full of questions, or resignation, or of worry about what the doctor or the nurse is going to say? And have you ever looked at the doctor's and the nurse's face to see how they respond to the patient's perception of them? Perception is a two-way operation. The weaker, more frightened and helpless we see the patient, the stronger, more confident and skilful we can feel ourselves to be. We can even be carried away by the patient's perception. We can feel so strong and clever and confident that we know best that we forget to listen to and look at the patient.

Up to a point, the patient may be perfectly happy with this state of affairs. He needs to see us as people who know best. 'It is common, inevitable and, indeed, important and useful, for the sick person to be able to surrender his adult independence and responsibility and to trust his fate to others' (Main, 1963). But here we get deep into the problem of communication between the sick who need help and the well who give it.

If we are so sure that we know best, and if our patients see us in that light, what kind of communication can there be between us? Our training and experience may give us the ability to meet their medical needs. In this area, we know best. That is why they come to us. But all we know of a patient's human needs is what we *believe* is best. We rarely ask him what he wants. If we get a patient who tells us, when we have not asked, we are taken aback. If he does not learn to behave according to our expectations he finds himself labelled 'uncooperative' (Schwartz, 1958), and removed to another ward or another hospital. Our belief that we know best is at once our strength and our weakness. On the one hand, it relieves the patient's anxiety and gives us the confidence to meet his medical needs; on the other, it can block communication. These attitudes are inherent in the system operated in the general hospital which is geared to meet the medical needs of patients. They themselves and their human needs, and we and our human needs take second place. In practice, these other considerations are often not in the running at all. We must first, last, and always get down to meeting medical needs. That is what a hospital is for.

The system, developed imperceptibly and without conscious planning, has, however, given rise to a number of problems now that we have remembered that medical and human needs are inseparable. How people feel towards each other, particularly towards those who are nearest to them or who are at the time most important to them, how they feel about their work and the life they lead, can affect their hearts, stomachs, lungs, and all the apparatus of their bodies. Family doctors and home nurses never forgot these facts of life, but in hospital we were absorbed in devising new techniques and discovering new therapeutic agents which revolutionized our ability to do our job, and in our justified absorption we tended to disregard human needs. Now that these have been reincorporated into medical science we can no longer do this. While it often seems to nurses that their medical colleagues in hospital are the least interested in patients as human beings and the most resistant to administrative changes to meet human needs, it is nevertheless true that these same colleagues have accelerated the changes by their own progress in medical science.

The dramatic advances of medicine during this century brought about other changes. Two of the most important of these are the rocketing cost of, and the enormous increase in public demand for, medical care in hospital. It became too expensive to be financed by the benevolence of the rich few or by the meagre funds of local authorities. Hospitals, no longer houses of death or of refuge for the destitute, became safe institutions which could pursue with increasing success a policy of active therapy for continually growing numbers of patients from all social classes. Towards the middle of this century, all medical care became a national responsibility in the United Kingdom. We witnessed fundamental changes in the ownership and management of hospitals. Every man and woman who works pays taxes, a portion of which (never enough, we feel) contributes to the upkeep and expansion of a national health service. The well pay for the care of the sick.

These changes in medicine itself and in the ownership and management of hospitals are creating far-reaching social changes in hospitals, which present us with fascinating new problems in nursing. We still have to nurse many of our sick in old forbidding institutions built for the elderly and orphaned destitute of a hundred years ago. We still dress ourselves up in slightly modified versions of the costumes of nineteenth-century chambermaids. Relics of nineteenth-century patronization of the deferential sick poor can still be detected in our attitudes to patients today. But people have realized that they are footing the bill and therefore have the right to a say in how they shall be treated. In typical fashion, in keeping with our national characteristic of demanding 'fair play', pressure groups are forming for this purpose. One aims to encourage or coerce maternity hospitals to 'humanize' their practices. Another has the same aim in general hospitals. These groups, regarded with mixed feelings by hospital authorities and staff, indicate something of what ordinary people are feeling about their treatment, and hospitals would be wise to take heed rather than umbrage. People know more about their bodies and about how sick bodies are made well. They are no longer content to lie back and let the doctors and nurses do it all. They want to know what is happening and to do their share. We, for our part, are learning how to use these attitudes as therapeutic tools. A patient who wants to know how to play his part in his own treatment makes our job more worth while and infinitely more interesting. But we are having to rethink ideas about how we work, how we see patients, the kind of setting we need for our job, and the kinds of conditions patients need in order to benefit from their stay with us.

If our assessment of patients' needs is based only on the belief that we know what is best for them, our thinking and subsequent planning may be sadly off-target. We have to put the belief to the test. We have to find out from patients themselves and to ask them in such a way that they can communicate their needs to us and will not feel that they must say what they believe we should like to hear.

It is only recently that we, in the United Kingdom and in Europe generally, have had any facts on which to base our discussion. We were forced to make up for this ignorance by falling back on our belief, and we are now only just beginning to find out if it is true or false. Testing belief is always a painful and upsetting process, as the reactions of nurses to some of the more penetrating studies have already shown. But research in all areas of hospital life is at last gathering momentum in the United Kingdom. We have begun to look at ourselves and to listen to patients with fresh eyes and ears. The first breakthrough in the study of patients' attitudes was made, perhaps naturally enough, in Scotland (McGhee, 1961). Similar studies were made in Lille, Rome, and other European centres at about the same time (Barnes, 1961; Ponzo and Meschieri, 1960; Sedes *et al.*, 1960). In 1963, for the first time, the Ministry of Health issued a 'List of Hospital Studies' a dozen or so of which are concerned, directly or indirectly, with hospital attitudes. With the help of the social scientists we are taking another look at this extraordinary social organization we thought we knew so well, questioning our ways of working in it and examining what it is doing to us and to our patients as human beings.

Happy, but potentially frustrating, signs of the times. Until the gap can be bridged between observation of problems and attempted solutions by changed administrative practices, until new practices are seen by everyone involved as changes for the better, and, perhaps most important, until social scientists and hospital staff can learn to understand each other's language, the research reports will remain just so much printed paper, and our discussion just so many lost words.

PART V

Summing Up

28 · Change as a Learning Situation[1]

BY DOREEN WEDDELL

To change the role of the nurse. This was the task that Dr Main and I set ourselves in 1946. We also sought to provide a training that would enable the anxieties unavoidable in nursing – concerning such matters as life and death, sex, psychosis, rage, despair – to be dealt with by methods other than those of distancing techniques and rigid non-personal hierarchies.

The events that I am reporting occurred during the seventeen years that I was the matron of the Cassel Hospital, and I am indebted to Dr Main and all who worked at the hospital with me in that period.

The medical aim was that life in hospital should reflect the ordinary living of patients, who should have responsibility, initiative, and freedom to go home as often as they could manage, while receiving psycho-analytically oriented psychotherapy.

The nursing staff came from general hospitals, for a year's course. They saw patients primarily as people for whom things had to be done. Families were usually rather a nuisance. The problem was how to enable the nurse to enjoy working with patients in ordinary household activities, welcoming family participation, while at the same time seeking to understand something of the whys and wherefores of the patients' disturbed relationships.

To achieve this, the work of the nurse was continually studied and redefined. Theoretical teaching was reduced and training occurred in seminar discussions about the nurses' experience in

[1] Reprinted from the 6th International Congress of Psychotherapy, London, 1964, *Psychotherapy and Psychosomatics*, Vol. 13, pp. 201–205, 1965 (S. Karger, Basel/New York); and from the *International Nursing Review*, Vol. 12, No. 5, 1965.

the ward. Each new nurse was attached to a more senior one, though each had her own group of patients with whom she worked.

There were three areas in which the nurse was constantly involved. One concerned the admission and discharge of patients and all the emotional upheaval of such events. The second centred on the disturbed behaviour of patients in various social settings, at home and at the hospital. The third concerned the observation of infants and young children in the hospital with their families.

The new nurse began by working with new patients, and it was not difficult for her to see how she shared with her patients some of the same problems of adjustment to a strange situation. Similarly, patients' problems about leaving hospital could be understood when linked to the nurse's own feelings about situations she had recently left.

The disturbances arising in the ward or community were examined as they occurred, with the people concerned. The question 'Who needs to get together with whom on this problem?' would begin the process of clarification. Attempts were made to understand the forces operating within and between groups in the hospital, in line with the ideas expressed by Main (1946, 1957),[1] Lewin (1947), Bion (1946, 1955, 1961), and Jaques (1951, 1955). The nurse came to recognize the manifestations of splitting and projection, scapegoating and pairing, significant in a group as well as for an individual. She could have the experience of the danger of suicide when a group was unconsciously vesting its murderousness in an individual; just as patients, or staff, might leave if they became the receptacles of a group's hostility. She would see how one ward or one group of patients, by projective identification, could stir up trouble or complain about another group or ward, in order to maintain a picture of themselves as having good relations with each other or their doctor. She might comprehend how, when two nurses were at loggerheads in the nursing group, it would not be long before this was reflected in the community behaviour of their patients. She might be able to see how she could come to feel that the medical staff were not doing their job, because that was what the patients were thinking. She would appreciate that she could be criticized by medical staff when they were feeling depressed or persecuted through their lack of success with some patients and needed a bad object, just as she might use

[1] See Chapters 1 and 5 – Ed.

patients for that purpose too. Something of the subtleties of the introjective and projective processes and something of her own defences could become clear to her, through the continuing attempt at understanding what might be going on in the community and the group.

It was in her work with infants and young children, in observing them at home, in the wards, in the nursery school, that the nurse obtained the conviction of the validity of the unconscious and the strength of infantile phantasy, and was able to recognize the 'child' still present inside herself, as in her patients. Constant discussion of these observations and possible meanings, in the vital emotional interplay between the child, his mother, his family, and herself, gave her an experience of significance, with internal meanings for herself as well as for her professional work.

With more understanding, patients as people became less frightening. The nurse became freer in herself, to take initiative and develop her own ideas, making it easier for patients to be allowed theirs. The recognition that the nurse also had feelings, that these could be noted and could be put to use in helping her to understand her patients, encouraged the recording of observations and the development of techniques of reporting. In perceiving what a patient might be doing to the nurse herself, or to the community, similar to what he had previously been doing to his family, the nurse could devise new ways of managing the situation.

From the beginning, a nurse could work with and seek to understand patients in very considerable states of disturbance, so long as there were acknowledged opportunities for relief for her, through discussion with other members of the staff, about every two to three hours. If these occasions were formalized, so that the nurse did not feel guilty at wanting this relief, then anxiety was reduced and a useful learning-teaching situation was available at the same time. For as long as the emotional experience was not too overwhelming, this was a situation in which learning could take place most easily. So, at least twice a day, sometimes more often, the nursing staff met together, not just to pass on information about patients or about doctors' wishes, but to examine what was going on and what they felt about it. An open discussion might then ensue on a particular patient or family, or on a community problem; or the discussion might focus on the future, anticipating events over the next week-end, for example.

I now give an instance of how, in such a setting, quite major changes in nursing role and technique came about. In the early days there were nurses on duty at night. At that time there were always several patients who did not sleep, and who would need the nurse, sometimes a doctor, occasionally a drug. When this situation was examined, it became clear that nurses who had perforce to be up at night also required patients to be awake and so to need them. The nurses themselves recognized their projection of dependency into the patients, and the patients' projection of competency into them. They decided to see what would happen if they went to bed at the same time as the patients did, around eleven o'clock. This idea was discussed with the patients who, though at first apprehensive, then thought it might be all right if they could be sure of having a nurse when they needed one and, significantly, if they could get up to get themselves cups of tea if they wanted to. For the patients, it became a situation in which they could assume a more adult role than the nurse would previously have allowed. For the nurse, the ward could become more like a household which would retire more or less at the same time, not necessarily being disturbed if one of its members was sleepless. In this context the nurse could easily understand something of a young child's Oedipal anxieties and conflicts, often most clearly expressed at bedtime. And, indeed, this method of nursing was dependent on the doctor who, though comfortably at home most of the time, could also be available to the nurse should she require him. It was not the disturbance caused by suicidal, murderous, or anxious patients that led her to call the doctor at night; nurses would deal with these upsets for weeks without undue difficulty; but if one of the medical staff was suspected of not being ready to support the nurse in her role, then there could be collapse of the nurses' morale, and requests for medical support became urgent and more frequent.

In conclusion, I should like to draw attention to a pattern of experience that occurred consistently over the years in the course of training nurses.

As a rule, when a new nurse came to the hospital she had high expectations of the working situation and of what she was going to learn. These lasted for about a month to six weeks. Then the idealization crumbled and the realities of awkward nurses, difficult patients, uninterested doctors intent on their own job, impinged. The nurse would long for the old hierarchies, for discipline, sureness, less responsibility for people. She would wish that she could again escape from people into practical tasks, be given instructions, be sure of diseases and cures. There might be panic and confusion at the lack of these things, because they served as defences (Menzies, 1960).

But, during the next four or five months, while continuing to experience and learn about a whole variety of situations, often with their own quite direct emotional impact, the nurse would be accomplishing a process of mourning within herself. She would be parting from previous ideals and known ways of thinking and behaving; questioning what she was learning; recognizing the value of ideas not thought of so highly before, rejecting some concepts, mulling over others, with some digestion going on.

Round about nine months from the beginning of the course, the nurse would begin to emerge from the confusion and depression, and begin to feel again some confidence in herself and in her skills. At this point she would have to start thinking about what she would do at the end of the course; how to make use of her new skills. She had to face problems of the unknown, with anticipation and anxiety, as anyone in such a situation. In other words, weaning experiences would again be revived: parting from friends, making new ones; regrets, disappointments, expectations; sifting, discarding, or storing ideas and memories; some idealization, some denigration. As at the beginning of the course, so at the end, such psychic work is an essential experience for the nurse, contributing to the understanding of herself and her patient.

Bibliography

BAKWIN, H. (1942). Loneliness in Infants. *American Journal of Diseases of Children* **63**, 30–40.

BALINT, M. (1952). On Love and Hate. In *Primary Love and Psycho-analytic Technique*. London: Hogarth. New edition, London: Tavistock Publications; New York: Liveright, 1965.

BALINT, M. (1957). *The Doctor, his Patient and the Illness*. London: Pitman.

BARNES, E. (1961). *People in Hospital*. London: Macmillan.

BENDER, L. and YARNELL, H. (1941). An Observation Nursery: A Study of 250 Children in the Psychiatric Division of Bellevue Hospital. *American Journal of Psychiatry* **97**, 1158–74.

BION, W. R. (1946). The Leaderless Group Project. *Bulletin of the Menninger Clinic* **10**, 3.

BION, W. R. (1955). Group Dynamics: A Review. In M. Klein, P. Heimann, R. E. Money-Kyrle (Eds.), *New Directions in Psycho-analysis*. London: Tavistock Publications.

BION, W. R. (1961). *Experiences in Groups*. London: Tavistock Publications; New York: Basic Books.

BOWLBY, J. (1946). *Forty-four Juvenile Thieves: their Characters and Home Life*. London: Baillière, Tindall & Cox.

BOWLBY, J. (1951). *Maternal Care and Mental Health*. Geneva: World Health Organization.

BRENMAN, M. (1952). On Teasing and Being Teased, and the Problem of 'Moral Masochism'. *Psychoanalytic Study of the Child* **7**, 246–85.

BURLINGHAM, D. and FREUD, A. (1942). *Young Children in Wartime: A Year's Experience in a Residential War Nursery*. London: Allen & Unwin.

BURLINGHAM, D. and FREUD, A. (1944). *Infants without Families*. London: Allen & Unwin; New York: International Universities Press.

CHAPIN, H. D. (1915). Are Institutions for Infants Necessary? *Journal of American Medical Association* **64,** 1–3.

ERIKSON, E. (1950). *Childhood and Society.* New York: Norton; London: Imago, 1951.

FREUD, A. (1937). *The Ego and the Mechanisms of Defence.* London: Hogarth.

FREUD, A. (1953). Some Remarks on Infant Observation. *Psychoanalytic Study of the Child* **8,** 9–19.

FREUD, S. (1900). *The Interpretation of Dreams. S.E.* Vols. 4 & 5, London: Hogarth, 1953.

FREUD, S. (1914). *Psychopathology of Everyday Life. S.E.* Vol. 6, London: Hogarth, 1960.

FREUD, S. (1921). *Group Psychology and the Analysis of the Ego. S.E.* Vol. 18, London: Hogarth, 1959.

GLUCK, I. and WRENN, M. (1959). Contribution to the Understanding of Disturbances of Mothering. *British Journal of Medical Psychology* **32,** 171–82.

GOLDFARB, W. (1943). Effects of Early Institutional Care on Adolescent Personality. *Journal of Experimental Education* **12,** 106–29.

GOLDFARB, W. (1944a). Effects of Early Institutional Care on Adolescent Personality: Rorschach Data. *American Journal of Orthopsychiatry* **14,** 441–7.

GOLDFARB, W. (1944b). Infant Rearing as a Factor in Foster Home Placement. *American Journal of Orthopsychiatry* **14,** 162–7.

GOLDFARB, W. and KLOPFER, B. (1944). Rorschach Characteristics of 'Institutional Children'. *Rorschach Research Exchange* **8,** 92–100.

IRVINE, R. E. and SMITH, B. J. (1963). Patterns of Visiting. *Lancet*, 16 March.

ISAACS, S. (1933). *Social Development of Young Children.* London: Routledge.

JAQUES, E. (1951). *The Changing Culture of a Factory.* London: Tavistock/Routledge.

JAQUES, E. (1955). Social Systems as a Defence against Persecutory and Depressive Anxiety. In M. Klein, P. Heimann, R. E. Money-Kyrle (Eds.), *New Directions in Psycho-analysis.* London: Tavistock Publications.

JONES, M. (1962). *Social Psychiatry in the Community, in Hospitals and in Prison.* Springfield, Illinois: C. C. Thomas.

KLEIN, M. (1932). *The Psycho-analysis of Children.* London: Hogarth.

KLEIN, M. (1946). Notes on Some Schizoid Mechanisms. In *Developments in Psycho-analysis.* London: Hogarth, 1952.

KLEIN, M. (1957). *Envy and Gratitude: A Study of Unconscious Sources.* London: Tavistock Publications.

KLEIN, M. (1959). Our Adult World and its Roots in Infancy. In *Our Adult World and Other Essays*. London: Heinemann, 1963.

KLEIN, M. and RIVIERE, J. (1936). *Love, Hate and Reparation.* Psycho-analyitcal Epitomes No. 2. London: Hogarth.

LEWIN, K. (1947). *Resolving Social Conflicts.* New York: Harper.

LOMAS, P. (1959). Husband-Wife Relationships in Cases of Puerperal Breakdown. *British Journal of Medical Psychology* **32,** 117.

LOMAS, P. (1960). Defensive Organization and Puerperal Breakdown. *British Journal of Medical Psychology* **33,** 61.

LOWREY, L. G. (1940). Personality Distortion and Early Institutional Care. *American Journal of Orthopsychiatry* **10,** 576–85.

MAIN, T. F. (1958). Mothers with Children in a Psychiatric Hospital. *Lancet*, 18 October, 845–7.

MAIN, T. F. (1963). Some Problems of Adaptation. *Physiotherapy*, May.

MCGHEE, A. (1961). *Patients' Attitudes to Nursing Care.* Edinburgh & London: Livingstone.

MELTZER, D. (1963). Dialogue with Adrian Stokes. In A. Stokes, *Painting and the Inner World.* London: Tavistock Publications.

MENZIES, I. E. P. (1960). A Case-study in the Functioning of Social Systems as a Defence against Anxiety: A Study of the Nursing Service of a General Hospital. *Human Relations* **13,** 95–121.

MINISTRY OF HEALTH (1947). Report of the Working Party on the Recruitment and Training of Nurses. London: HMSO.

MINISTRY OF HEALTH (1948). Minority Report of the Working Party on the Recruitment and Training of Nurses, by John Cohen. London: HMSO.

MINISTRY OF HEALTH (1961). Report of the Sub-committee on the Pattern of the In-Patient's Day (Chairman: M. B. Powell, DBE). Central Health Services Council. London: HMSO.

MINISTRY OF HEALTH (1963). List of Hospital Studies. HM(63)18. London: HMSO.

MINISTRY OF HEALTH (1966). Report of the Committee on Senior Nursing Staff Structure (Chairman: Mr B. Salmon). London: HMSO.

MONEY-KYRLE, R. E. (1956). Normal Counter-transference and Some of its Deviations. *International Journal of Psycho-Analysis* **37,** 360–6.

MONEY-KYRLE, R. E. (1961). *Man's Picture of his World.* London: Duckworth.

PONZO, E. and MESCHIERI, L. (1960). Atteggiamenti e razioni dei pazienti degli ospedali generali. Estratto dalla *Rassegna di Psicologia Generale e Clinica*, Anno 5, Vol. 5, Fasc. 3, Settembre-Diciembre.

REVANS, R. W. (1960). The Hospital as an Organism: A Study of Communications and Morale. In *Proceedings of the 6th International Meeting of the Institute of Management Sciences*, held in Paris, 1959. Oxford: Pergamon.

RIBBLE, M. (1943). *The Rights of Infants*. New York: Columbia University Press.

RIDLEY, U. (1956). *The Babies' Hospital*. Newcastle-on-Tyne: Reid.

ROGERSON, C. H., HARDCASTLE, D. H., and DUGUID, K. (1935). A Psychological Approach to the Problem of Asthma and the Asthma-Eczema-Purigo Syndrome. *Guy's Hospital Reports*, Vol. 85, No. 3 (Vol. 15, Fourth Series).

ROSS, T. A. (1923). *The Common Neurosis*. London: Edward Arnold.

ROSS, T. A. (1932). *An Introduction to Analytic Psychotherapy*. London: Edward Arnold.

ROSS, T. A. (1936). *An Enquiry into the Prognosis of Neurosis*. Cambridge: Cambridge University Press.

SCHWARTZ, D. (1958). 'Uncooperative' Patients. *American Journal of Nursing* **58**, No. 1.

SEDES, J. M., AUREL, C., DESTOMBES, A., and NAYRAC, P. (1960). Étude psycho-sociologique à la cité hospitalière de Lille. (Unpublished paper.)

SEGAL, H. (1952). A Psycho-analytical Approach to Aesthetics. *International Journal of Psycho-Analysis* **33**, 190–207.

SEGAL, H. (1957). Notes on Symbol Formation. *International Journal of Psycho-Analysis* **38**, 391–7.

SINGEISEN, F. (1960). Problèmes psychologiques à l'hôpital général. *Médecine et Hygiène* **18**.

SPENCE, J. C. (1946). Nurseries and the Welfare of Children. *Journal of the Royal Sanitary Institute* **66**, 323–6.

SPITZ, R. A. (1945). Hospitalism: An Inquiry into the Genesis of Psychiatric Conditions in Early Childhood. *Psychoanalytic Study of the Child* **1**, 53–74.

SPITZ, R. A. (1946). Hospitalism: A Follow-up Report. *Psychoanalytic Study of the Child* **2**, 113–17.

SPITZ, R. A. (1947). Emotional Growth in the First Year. *Child Study*, Spring.

SPITZ, R. A. (1950). Psychiatric Therapy in Infancy. *American Journal of Orthopsychiatry* **20**, 623–33.

SPITZ, R. A. and WOLF, K. M. (1946). Anaclitic Depression: An Inquiry into the Genesis of Psychiatric Conditions in Early Childhood. *Psychoanalytic Study of the Child* **2**, 313–42.

SPITZ, R. A. and WOLF, K. M. (1949). Autoerotism: Some Empirical Findings and Hypotheses on Three of its Manifestations in the First Year of Life. *Psychoanalytic Study of the Child* **3/4**, 85–120.

STANTON, A. H. and SCHWARTZ, M. S. (1949a). The Management of a

Type of Institutional Participation in Mental Illness. *Psychiatry* **12**, 13–26.

STANTON, A. H. and SCHWARTZ, M. S. (1949b). Medical Opinion and the Social Context in the Mental Hospital. *Psychiatry* **12**, 243–9.

STANTON, A. H. and SCHWARTZ, M. S. (1949c). Observations on Dissociation as Social Participation. *Psychiatry* **12**, 339–54.

STANTON, A. H. and SCHWARTZ, M. S. (1954). *The Mental Hospital*. New York: Basic Books.

WEDDELL, D. (1955). Psychology Applied to Nursing. A series of 'Notes' for tutors and others concerned in the training of student nurses. *Nursing Times*, September 1954–March 1955. Also reprinted as a pamphlet.

WINNICOTT, D. W. (1957a). *The Child and the Family*. London: Tavistock Publications.

WINNICOTT, D. W. (1957b). *The Child and the Outside World*. London: Tavistock Publications.

WINNICOTT, D. W. (1965). *The Family and Individual Development*. London: Tavistock Publications; New York: Basic Books.

FILMS

GLUCK, I. and WRENN, M. (1960). *Play and Personality*. Cassel Hospital, Richmond, Surrey. Also available from New York University Film Library, and Edric Films Ltd, Gerrards Cross, Bucks.

ROBERTSON, J. (1953). *A Two-Year-Old Goes to Hospital*. London: Tavistock Child Development Research Unit; New York; New York University Film Library.

SPITZ, R. A. (1946). *Grief: A Peril in Infancy*. New York: New York University Film Library. Also available from the Cassel Hospital, Richmond, Surrey.

Index